LOVE LIFE -

Riki Davies

Cover image licensed from 123RF Stock Photos

ISBN: 978-1-61364-909-1

Dedication

This book is dedicated to my son, Johnathan, who for the past 19 years has been my joy and inspiration.

Acknowledgments

My most abundant gratitude goes to my wonderful friend Christine Mitchell-Bond for her total support and faith in me, her help and encouragement, and belief that I can write this book so that others can discover the true path to good health.

CONTENTS

Understanding the Benefits of Healthy Eating

We are all used to hearing how we should eat healthily, exercise more and cut down our stress levels to maintain a healthy body but what does healthy eating really mean to the average person – the man or woman trying to overcome a serious illness or lose weight? One of the latest recommendations is that we have 5-7 portions of fruit and vegetables a day and eat smaller portions at meals – but smaller portions of what, precisely?

Healthy eating applies to ALL the foods and drinks we consume. Unknowingly, many of us are eating foods that are harmful, causing inflammation and allowing a host of other irritants to attack our bodies, leaving us tired and drained or physically ill. No-one should have to go through life feeling unwell and not understand why.

After working for several years within the Macmillan cancer support organisation and interacting with patients on a regular basis, I began looking for other ways in which I could contribute to their recovery. Being a medical herbalist with a considerable knowledge of nutrition, I began writing down all that I had discovered throughout years of research. I had come to believe that looking at diet from the inside out is vital to better health, not only for cancer patients but for anyone suffering from severe to even minor conditions. Being a volunteer at Macmillan via the NHS, I was not allowed to use my expertise to give diet advice; therefore I am writing this book, which contains recipes for healing and nourishing the body, along with sound nutritional advice to help raise awareness amongst those seeking to find the way forward to a healthier, more revitalized life.

Whilst the recipes I have selected for this book are not based on raw foods, I am a great believer in eating most foods as nature creates them. This is because cooked foods trigger an immune response in the body that raw foods do not. What the body does is to inundate the blood with white blood cells, which means the body is preparing itself to battle against infection and foreign materials (the cooked foods!). However, by eating a mainly raw food diet there is little or no infection and, consequently, fewer white blood cells.

You may also find that you need less sleep. It is during sleep that the body does most of its healing. Therefore, the more the body is abused with cooked foods or stress, the more time it needs to heal itself. If you take away the cause of abuse, you may not only sleep less but the sleep that you do have will be more refreshing and revitalizing.

However, I am fully aware that not everyone can tolerate raw foods or enjoy eating totally cold foods. I only suggest that, where possible, you give it a try and feel its benefits. If it is definitely not for you, try lightly steaming your food but be careful – NEVER OVERCOOK!

So please take time to read and 'digest' the following information and refer to it from time to time in your quest for a healthier, fitter you.

Dehydrating food

Dehydrating food is essential for today's raw food enthusiasts. It is a way of preserving fruits, vegetables, nuts and herbs for use at a later date, conserving their nutritional value and concentrating flavours. It also ensures that moulds and yeasts are unable to grow on the food and spoil it.

Food dehydration can be carried out in a fan-assisted oven or even outside in the sun. However, when food is cooked at temperatures above 48°C many of its essential nutrients are destroyed. Also, subjecting foods to high temperatures leaves it hard on the outside but still moist in the middle, which can still allow mould to form. However, an electric food dehydrator with a variable temperature regulator (which starts as low as 29°C) gives the user more control and produces the best results.

The benefits of food dehydration

- Control the quality of the food you eat. Dehydrated foods are delicious, nutritious, easy to prepare, easy to use, and easily carried in lunch-packs.
- Save money. Unlike canned or packet foods, when containers of dehydrated foods are opened and closed again there will be no harmful effects on the contents.
- Make the most of seasonal foods. By dehydrating seasonal foods from your garden or the supermarket you will be able to use them for much longer.
- Take advantage of special offers at the supermarket.

- Create your own food supply. With dehydrated foods available, there are always ingredients to rely on when money gets tight.
- Help the environment. By dehydrating your own foods, you are cutting down on packaging.

How to store dehydrated foods

Dehydrated foods should always be stored in airtight containers and labelled with the contents and date. Store the containers in a dry, dark place with a moderate temperature, e.g. your kitchen cupboard or pantry. Dried foods will last approximately one year in airtight containers. If dehydrated foods are kept for longer than a year, they will begin to darken in colour and lose their flavour. Therefore, please remember to date the foods and to use the oldest first.

Eat foods that are rich in nutrients

Nutrient-rich foods naturally contain one or more of the following:

- Vitamins
- Minerals
- Enzymes
- Healthy protein
- Healthy fat (including cholesterol)
- Healthy carbohydrates (including fibre)
- Phytonutrients (from plant foods)
- Water

Dark or brightly coloured vegetables, fruits, and legumes are nature's most nutrient-rich plant foods and are well-tolerated by most people. Free-range eggs and cold-water fish are good nutrient-rich foods though, for some, eggs can be hard to digest.

Soups made from vegetables, cold-water fish or organic chickens (including the bones) are all excellent nutritional choices.

Avoid highly processed foods

Highly processed foods have very little nutritional value. So try to avoid sugar, flour and highly processed grains, such as those found in many ready-made breakfast cereals. Deep-fried foods like crisps also lack nutrients and are wasted calories.

Highly processed foods may not be injurious to your body in the short term if your health is reasonably good but by avoiding this group of foods altogether you will be healthier both in the short and long term.

Chew your foods well

As discussed above, a vital principle to eating healthily is to consume nutrient-rich foods. Vegetables, fruits, beans, peas, lentils, nuts, and eggs are good examples of health-promoting, nutrient-rich foods. However, eating them in a hurry (or worse still – on the run) is not the way to good health.

Thoroughly chewing your foods until they take a more liquid form eases the burden on the digestive organs and helps the body to extract and absorb the maximum amount of nutrients from your foods. Remember to chew each mouthful at least 30 times for ease of digestion and good health.

Avoid foods that cause cellular injury or inflammation

According to research on health and nutrition, the worst culprits for causing damage to the body are:

- dairy products (with the exception of live yogurt)
- sugar
- salt (use vegetable salt, in moderation, as an alternative)
- foods containing shortening or partially hydrogenated oils
- highly processed bacon, luncheon meats and sausages
- over-cooked factory-farmed meats (e.g. barbecuing)
- fizzy drinks.

These foods should be avoided.

Eating well

Breakfast:

- Some type of fruit – and eat an apple often
- Make juices – see **Juices** on page 61
- Make smoothies – see **Smoothies** on page 53
- From time to time make green juice such as lettuce, celery or wheatgrass – see **Grow Your Own Wheatgrass** on page 286

- Boiled or scrambled egg mixed with almond/rice or coconut milk – see **Make Your Own Almond Milk** on page 50
- Healthy cereal made with almond, rice or hazelnut milk
- Porridge with almond milk, cinnamon and either blueberries or, if you need to sweeten it, a small amount of Manuka honey or Stevia granules (in cases of severe health problems I would recommend you use blueberries only)
- Chlorella – see **Sun chlorella** on pages 285; 319
- Vitamin D3 5000 IU (in winter).

Lunch:

- Bowl of vegetable and pulse soup (cold or warm)
- Steamed vegetables or salad based on plenty of in-season green salad, pulses, seeds and nuts
- Organic brown rice, quinoa
- Vegetable pâté with bite size pieces of celery, carrot and cucumber
- Cold-water fish such as organic salmon, sardines, tuna, trout, haddock and mackerel.

Dinner:

- A mix of pulses
- Quinoa and vegetables steamed or lightly boiled
- Hummus/tahini paste (freshly made)

- Meals of vegetables and pulses are best for optimal health, but if you must eat meat then organic chicken is a better choice of protein consumption than red meat.

Snacks:

If you want a snack then try to base it on the following:

- A variety of nuts such as almonds, cashews, brazil nuts, walnuts etc
- Hemp or almond butter is a good, nutritious spread
- Smoothies – see **Smoothies** on page 53
- Fresh coconut is a good snack and quite filling
- Shredded raw vegetables such as carrots, cucumber, celery etc, would be a good choice to promote a healthy gut
- Goji berries.

Try to base your meals mainly on organic raw foods when possible.

Getting the most out of what you eat

For the body to thrive we need not only to eat a good variety of foods but in different forms.

Fresh leafy green vegetables and salad greens, when eaten raw, provide a wealth of vitamins, minerals, enzymes, fibre, water and phytonutrients. However, they do have a tough fibrous content and can be difficult to chew thoroughly enough to optimally extract the nutrients.

We all need to eat our leafy green vegetables in order to promote good overall health, and eating them in a variety of forms (cooked or raw) will ensure that we get the best from them.

For instance:

- Juicing a head of romaine lettuce, parsley and/or coriander leaves releases all of the goodness in the lettuce, ensuring that your body has easy access to its health-giving nutrients.

- Steaming or boiling (for as short a time as possible!) will soften the fibre in vegetables, especially vegetables such as cabbage and carrots. Although some heat-sensitive nutrients might be lost in the process, the benefits gained from eating the vegetables far outweigh any losses.

When boiling vegetables, why not use the water as a base for soups as it will contain some of the nutrients from the vegetables?

Homemade soups are full of nutrients that are easily absorbed and essential to developing and maintaining healthy bones, teeth, nerve and muscle function.

Homemade soups are nourishing and will not damage the health like dairy products (often the principal ingredient in many recipes); the risk of developing any health problems associated with regular dairy intake – sinus infections, a blocked nose, ear infections, diarrhoea, bloody stools, stomach cramps, skin disorders such as eczema, immune system failure and more – can be greatly reduced and even eliminated by eating homemade soups instead of dairy products.

To make vegetable soup, see **Soups** on page 97. If you wish to use organic chicken, use the same method and just add the chicken, including some bones for their micronutrients.

The benefit of pulses

Peas and beans belong to a family of vegetables called pulses. They are packed with complex carbohydrate, and are an inexpensive source of low-fat fibre, protein and minerals. Chickpeas assist adrenal function and are rich in protein, EFAs and iron; lentils are rich in protein and iron and help support the heart and kidneys; while soya beans are full of nutrients such as protein, EFAs and lecithin. Soya also contains a natural source of oestrogen, which is invaluable for women nearing the menopause.

For optimum nutrition, eat pulses twice a day. Try different pulses such as aduki beans, black-eyed peas, mung beans, kidney, lima, or cannellini beans, in stews and salads or on their own as a snack.

Green vegetables can strengthen your heart

Studies have shown that eating green vegetables regularly can not only reduce the risk of having a heart attack but also boost your chances of survival by up to a third should you have an attack. This is thanks to nitrite, a healing component found in high quantities in most green vegetables. The benefits come from nitrite's conversion to nitric oxide when oxygen levels drop during an attack. Nitric oxide widens the arteries, increasing the supply of oxygen to the heart.

Should raw foods be eaten in cold weather?

The advantages of eating raw foods are numerous. Fruits, vegetables, nuts and seeds are full of natural goodness and, eaten raw, are undamaged by heating and processing. There are, however, disadvantages to eating nothing but raw foods. They are not always easy to digest as the fibres have not been softened enough by heating. Light cooking can also make some of the nutrients more available and therefore more easily absorbed by the body. However, in winter, it is without doubt better for the body to stay well-warmed with lightly cooked foods. Steaming foods is an excellent way of cooking as the nutrients are left intact. I recommend that you change the balance of raw to cooked food according to the season. Try a combination of raw and cooked foods in winter and eat more raw foods in the warmer months. Where possible, always choose organic fruits and vegetables that are in season, and if you can grow your own – all the better.

The acid-alkaline (pH) balance

How many times have we all read about the importance of preserving the correct acid-alkaline balance in our bodies? Just what are we supposed to do with this information? Even more problematic is finding out whether we're acid or alkaline to start with. What follows is a simple explanation of what the pH balance is and how we can ensure the perfect balance for our bodies.

pH (i.e. the potential of hydrogen) is the measure of hydrogen ions in a given solution. For the layman, that tells us how acid or alkaline something is on a scale of 0 to 14, with 0 being extremely acid, 14 being extremely alkaline and 7 being neutral.

Human blood has a pH value ranging between 7.3 and 7.45. Anything under a pH of 5.5 can have an adverse effect on the body. Since blood nourishes all of our organs and tissues, it is essential that we maintain its alkaline pH. We can do this chiefly via the foods we eat.

Unfortunately the foods that most people eat today are processed and/or full of chemicals, which results in them being highly acidic. To put it simply, most of the foods available today are injurious to our health and should not even be considered when planning meals.

Also, knowing which foods are acidic is not as easy as it sounds. Those that test acidic in a laboratory (such as lemons) are actually very alkalizing in the body. Another problem is that we often combine foods and unwittingly create too much acid in the body.

If we have too much acid in our bodies, our organs cannot function properly. We can start to feel aches and pains while diseases flourish; premature ageing can gather pace; and excess weight can pile on – all practically guaranteed to either shorten or devastate our lives.

Looking on the bright side, the ideal acid-alkaline balance is easy to accomplish and sustain by following the 3 steps below:

1. Eat a diet of at least 70% alkaline foods and combine all of your meals carefully.

2. Drink pure water (at least 5-8 cups a day). Try adding a little freshly-squeezed lemon juice to make it more alkaline. Remember – pure water; this does not include the water contained in coffee, tea, fizzy or sweetened drinks.

3. Check your pH on a regular basis. You can get a self-test kit online; however, a blood test carried out by a doctor is the most accurate test available.

Alkaline foods

Vegetables: Artichokes, asparagus, beetroot, broccoli, brussels sprouts, cabbage, carrot, cauliflower, celery, chives, courgette, cucumber, garlic, grasses (wheat, straw, barley, etc), green beans, kale, lamb's lettuce, leeks, lettuce, onion, peas, radish, red cabbage, spinach, swede, turnip, watercress.

Fruits: Avocado, grapefruit, lemon, lime, rhubarb, tomato, watermelon.

Drinks: Green drinks, fresh vegetable juice, pure water (distilled or ionised), lemon water (pure water with fresh lemon or lime), vegetable broth, non-sweetened soya milk, almond milk, herbal teas.

Seeds, Nuts & Grains: Almonds, any sprouted seed, buckwheat, cumin seeds, flax, lentils, pumpkin, sesame, spelt, sunflower.

Fats & Oils: Flax, hemp, avocado, olive, evening primrose, borage, coconut oil, oil blends.

Others: Hummus, sprouts, (alfalfa, broccoli, chickpea, mung bean, little radish, soya, wheat, etc), tahini.

Acid foods

Meats: Beef, chicken, crustaceans, lamb, other seafood (apart from occasional oily fish such as salmon), pork, turkey.

Dairy Products: Cheese, cream, eggs, ice cream, milk, yogurt.

Others: Artificial sweeteners, biscuits, condiments (mayonnaise, tomato sauce, etc), honey, soy sauce, tamari, vinegar, white bread, white pasta, wholemeal bread.

Drinks: Beers, coffee, dairy smoothies, fizzy drinks, fruit juice, milk, spirits, tea, traditional tea.

Convenience Foods: Chocolate, fast food, instant meals, microwave meals, powdered soups, sweets, tinned foods.

Fats & Oils: Corn oil, hydrogenated oils, margarine, saturated fats, sunflower oil, vegetable oil.

Fruits: All fruits apart from those listed as alkaline.

Seeds & Nuts: Cashew nuts, peanuts, pistachio nuts.

Antioxidants

One of the best ways to help prohibit Alzheimer's, Parkinson's disease, cancer and heart disease, is by consuming plenty of antioxidant-rich foods. Antioxidants help prevent and repair damage in the body caused by free radicals.

Antioxidants are most abundant in brightly coloured plant foods. The highest calibre antioxidant-rich foods in the four main food groups are as follows:

Fruits	Vegetables	Nuts	Spices
blueberries	beans	pecans	cinnamon
cranberries	artichoke hearts	walnuts	oregano
blackberries	russet potatoes	hazelnuts	ground cloves

Aim to eat plenty of fresh vegetables daily, either raw or juiced. But always remember to thoroughly wash any non-organic fruits and vegetables first to eradicate harmful pesticides.

Calcium

We're all aware that calcium can help us avoid osteoporosis, but how many of us realize that calcium is also needed by the body to help the heart and metabolism to function at optimum levels? Read on to find out how getting sufficient calcium can improve your health.

Calcium can help with weight control: When the body lacks sufficient calcium, it goes into emergency mode and releases parathyroid hormone into the system. This, in turn, stimulates the bones to release calcium into the blood stream, and the kidneys to release a hormone called calcitrol (a form of vitamin D), which boosts the body's capacity to absorb calcium.

Unfortunately, these two hormones also stimulate the production of fat and impede its breakdown; ergo, the body stores fat and stubbornly holds on to it, even if a low-calorie diet is adopted.

However, a high intake of calcium inhibits the parathyroid and calcitrol hormones, causing the body to store less fat and also to break it down easily.

Calcium helps protect your heart: Researchers believe that those of us who are low on calcium are more likely to have high blood pressure. When the body releases calcitrol in response to a calcium shortage, it constricts the smooth muscle walls of the arteries, thereby elevating blood pressure.

So our calcium intake may be almost as important in the case of blood pressure as our intake of sodium. A sufficient supply of calcium encourages the muscles (including the heart muscle) to efficiently contract and relax (see **How much calcium do I need?** on page 17).

Calcium – a protection against colon cancer? Researchers believe that an adequate intake of calcium could reduce the risk of colon cancer. Although it's not clear why this happens, it is believed that the excess calcium left in the stomach, after the body has taken what it needs, binds with cancer promoters and are passed out of the body together.

Calcium protects the teeth: A lack of calcium affects our teeth in a roundabout way – that's because the calcium in our teeth usually stays put. So why should we concern ourselves? Well, actually it's the jawbone that's the problem here. Just like other bones, it gives up calcium for the body's needs when there's a lack. And as the jawbone deteriorates, the teeth loosen and become a breeding ground for bacteria, causing infection, inflammation and bleeding.

Calcium-rich foods

Yogurt (live); orange juice, calcium-fortified; sardines, canned (with bones); wild salmon, canned (with bones); soya milk, calcium-fortified; sesame seeds; kale, cooked; tofu with calcium sulphate; blackstrap molasses; white beans, cooked; figs, dried; quinoa, cooked; broccoli, raw or cooked; spinach, cooked; rhubarb, cooked; red beans, cooked.

It's important we get the bulk of our calcium from foods, in order to benefit from the other nutrients they provide. It is widely believed that low-fat or non-fat dairy products, including yogurt and milk, are an ideal way to get calcium. However, dairy consumption is a contentious subject (see **Milk** on page 18).

How much calcium do I need?

Ages 9 to 18	1,300 mg a day
Ages 19 to 50	1,000 mg a day
Ages 51 and above	1,200 mg a day

Calcium supplements

- Aim to get your daily amount of calcium from a combination of food and supplements and avoid consuming more than 2,500 mg a day in supplement form; as this could increase the risk of kidney stones.

- Avoid taking more than 500 mg of calcium supplements at any one time as the body cannot absorb a whole day's supply in one go.

- It is also advisable to take one dose at night to replenish the calcium lost from the bones as you sleep.

- Taking vitamin D supplements helps the body to effectively absorb calcium

- If you have hyperparathyroidism or a history of kidney stones, you should consult a doctor before taking calcium supplements.

Milk

How many times have we heard 'nutritional experts' singing the praises of cow's milk? So much so, that we give it to our children to ensure they have strong teeth and healthy bones. But are we really doing our best for them by giving them what nature actually intended for baby cows? A new-born calf weighing 80-100 lbs will end up weighing approximately 550 lbs when fully weaned – and all due to its mother's milk! Cow's milk contains 300 times more casein than human milk. Casein is a glutinous substance that encourages the formation of huge cow bones. But when consumed by a human, it's almost impossible to digest and is acid forming in the stomach.

Research has shown a link between the consumption of milk and other dairy products to many of the most common diseases in the world today – heart disease, cancer, arthritis, migraines, allergies, asthma, etc – all disorders that can be caused or worsened by acid.

Cow's milk, like other dairy products, coats the mucus membranes, causing a build-up of dense, slow-moving mucus. So if you or your children seem to have constant runny noses and/or earaches, try eliminating milk and other dairy foods from your diet for a month or so. It's certainly a better option than frequent antibiotics from your G.P.

Fortunately, milk and other dairy products are not essential to get calcium (see **Calcium**, on page 15).

An excellent substitute for cow's milk is almond milk. Almond milk is simple to make in a blender from raw almonds, plus a few dates if you prefer your milk slightly sweeter; see my recipe for **Almond milk** on page 50.

Water

The human body is made up of over 70% water, every drop of which is vital for the body and its organs to function properly. It is crucial for digestion, absorption, circulation and excretion by helping to carry nutrients in and out of cells, expelling waste and maintaining a normal body temperature.

Most of us do not drink enough water – we should all aim to drink 6-8 glasses a day. Hot water with a slice of lemon and herbal teas count towards your water intake, but other drinks do not.

Soft and carbonated drinks

'Soft drinks' is the name given to beverages that are free from alcohol. They are much favoured by the younger generation, many of whom would prefer to drink a can of 'pop' rather than a glass of pure water.

However, they are particularly harmful to health and should be avoided. To understand fully what they contain, and the harm they can do to the body, read on.

Caffeine

Whilst caffeine may improve the flavour of fizzy drinks, it is an addictive drug that stimulates the nervous system and increases the heart rate. Upon consumption, the drinker may feel more alert and experience a temporary boost in brain power.

However, over-stimulation saps the body of vital energy as it attempts to deal with the toxin that enters the bloodstream. High caffeine consumption has been linked to bladder and stomach cancer, raised blood pressure and aggravation of diabetes symptoms.

Sugar

Most soft drinks contain up to 15 teaspoons of refined sugar in each 325 ml can – more than a whole day's recommended allowance. The GDA given on labels for 'total sugars' (sugars added to foods plus those that occur naturally, e.g. in fruit) for women is 90g, and 120g for men, but everyone should aim to consume less than 50g of 'added sugar' per day.

Sugar damages our teeth as well as increasing the risk of heart disease and diabetes. Unfortunately, the more sugar we consume, the more the body craves it – a dependency that is hard to break.

Artificial sweeteners

Diet sodas contain artificial sweeteners such as acesulfame-k, aspartame and saccharin. These calorie-reduced sweeteners are used as an alternative to sugar – hence the 'diet' aspect. However:

Acesulfame-K is 100-200 times sweeter than sugar, with a slight bitter aftertaste. Preliminary tests suggest that this substance may be carcinogenic. Even though tests are ongoing, it would be advisable to refrain from ingesting acesulfame-k as laboratory animals have shown a rapid increase in cancerous tumours.

Aspartame (also known as AminoSweet or Senomyx) is 200 times sweeter than sugar, and whilst it improves the taste of the drink, it can also trigger a variety of adverse side-effects. Among the most commonly reported medical problems are blurred vision, emotional disorders, heart palpitations, memory loss, migraine, ringing in the ears and shortness of breath.

Saccharin is a calorie-free sweetener and is 300-450 times sweeter than sugar. Some people experience a bitter or metallic aftertaste when consuming products containing this substance. When tested on rats they developed bladder cancer. It has been banned in Canada, New Zealand and several European countries.

Acids

Citric, tartaric and phosphoric acids are used in the majority of soft drinks and are added to give them their familiar tang, whilst conserving their sweetness. But don't be fooled – they can burn your insides.

An acidic gut is an ideal environment for many diseases to flourish, whilst an acidic blood condition can undermine the immune system.

Whilst some cells die in an acidic environment, others attempt to adapt in order to survive and become abnormal malignant cells.

Carbon dioxide

The making of fizzy drinks involves injecting carbon dioxide into water under pressure to make it bubbly.

The human body treats carbon dioxide as a waste product, exhaling it from the lungs, and it beggars belief that we are expected to take it into our bodies in the form of drinks. Excessive carbon dioxide can kill healthy cells, and these dead cells trigger an acidic environment, which, as we have already seen, can be extremely harmful to the body.

Sodium

Inorganic sodium is added to most soft drinks. It is used as an emulsifying, stabilizing and thickening agent to keep the various contents of the drinks evenly distributed. An excessive dietary consumption of inorganic sodium also thickens and stiffens the arteries, which can lead to high blood pressure, strokes, cardiac failure, some forms of kidney disease, PMT and many other ailments.

Preservatives

Preservatives are added to soft drinks to prevent spoilage and to extend their shelf life. Both storage conditions and time can affect the flavour of the drinks and preservatives help to prevent that happening.

While labels may list the following as permitted preservatives, an excessive amount can cause many serious health problems.

Sodium benzoate (benzoic acid) is a chemical used in most soft drinks and is known to cause asthma, rashes and hyperactivity.

Sulphur dioxide, although not as commonly used, is present in some soft drinks. It is important to remember that this chemical is also used for industrial bleaching and is so toxic that repeated exposures can cause fainting spells, skin eruptions, swelling, tightening of the chest, shock, coma and death.

Artificial flavourings and colourings

Artificial flavourings are commonly added to soft drinks to give each its own characteristic taste. However, they can have an adverse effect on children who are hyperactive and therefore must be eliminated from their diet.

Tartrazine is a yellow food and drink colouring that is produced synthetically from petroleum. The use of tartrazine is banned in Norway and Finland, and was also banned in Austria and Germany until the ban was overturned by a European Union directive. In April 2008, the United Kingdom's Food Standards Agency called for a voluntary phase-out of tartrazine along with five other colourings, due to a reported link with hyperactivity in children. It can cause allergic reactions like skin disorders, swelling, respiratory problems, excessive mucus and bloodshot eyes.

Carmoisine is a red food and drink colouring that is banned in the USA and other countries, but permitted for use in the UK. It can cause allergic reactions, food poisoning and even cancer.

Brilliant blue is another cancer-causing agent that has been certified as a safe food additive in the EU. This chemical can cause chromosomal damage and allergic reactions.

Coffee and tea

Coffee is highly addictive. You drink coffee in the morning to wake you up and give a boost of energy; however, within a few hours your energy levels plummet, which makes you want another coffee. This cycle continues until your body becomes totally dependent on coffee to function properly throughout the day. This rise and fall in the body's energy levels is what feeds the addiction.

The fallacy that the bad effects of coffee (increased energy and heightened mental ability followed by fatigue, irritability, sleeplessness, heartburn and ulcers) are caused by caffeine alone is a misconception. There are 500 or more chemicals in coffee, many of which are harmful to the body. Coffee is also a crop with high pesticide residues including Aldrin, Chlordane, Dieldrin and Heptachlor (all banned for use within the EU), a fact that has lead some experts to say that coffee beans are one of the major sources of toxins that we consume every day.

Black tea and coffee have a lot in common, although they are different plants and come from different parts of the world. Tea contains caffeine and other members of the same drug family, methyl xanthines. Tea also contains tannin, which is used as a tanning agent. If consumed in excessive quantities, tannins inhibit the absorption of minerals such as iron which may, if prolonged, lead to anaemia. Adding lemon juice to tea will reduce the negative effect of tannins in iron absorption as well, while adding milk to tea has very little or no influence on the effect of tannins.

In sensitive individuals, a large intake of tannins may cause bowel irritation, kidney irritation, liver damage, irritation of the stomach and gastrointestinal pain.

Green teas are the mildest of the caffeine drinks and have beneficial phytochemicals, which makes their use a more attractive option than other teas and coffees.

Salt and sodium

The difference between salt and sodium

Salt is not sodium; however, it does contain high levels of sodium. Table salt consists of 40% sodium and 60% chloride. Regular table salt has 2,350 mg sodium per teaspoon, while sea salt's sodium content is almost as high at 2,132mg per teaspoon.

Salt and the human body

We all need a daily intake of salt (sodium chloride) as it cannot be reproduced by the body. Salt is needed by the human body to help muscles and nerves to work and to regulate blood pressure. Hormones help the body regulate how much salt and water is needed.

However, the body loses salt through urine, perspiration, vomiting and diarrhoea. If too much salt is lost, the level of fluid in the blood will drop, so we do need a small amount to maintain a healthy body.

Salt is often used as a preservative and is added to most processed and pre-packaged foods. If you add salt when you cook, this greatly increases your intake. However, for optimal health, the recommended daily amount of salt is 6g. Unfortunately, this is easily exceeded – the average salt intake in the UK being 9-12g per day.

The dangers of excessive sodium intake

A high sodium intake has also been linked to other conditions, such as:

- Gastric cancer
- Heart failure
- Kidney problems and kidney stones
- Left ventricular hypertrophy
- Oedema
- Stroke

A high level of salt intake increases the amount of calcium expelled in the urine, which may also contribute to osteoporosis.

Many foods today purport to be reduced salt or low salt but this can be confusing when labels refer only to sodium. To calculate the amount of salt in a food, multiply the sodium content on the label by 2.5. *Remember, you should aim to consume no more than 6g of salt a day.*

As for your own home-cooked food, why not consider replacing salt with tasty herbs and spices?

Chocolate

Chocolate is a psychoactive food that acts primarily upon the central nervous system where it alters brain function, resulting in changes in perception, mood, consciousness and behaviour. One of the methyl xanthine drugs, theobromine, is found in chocolate as well as coffee and tea. This drug is related to caffeine.

It is the drugs in the cocoa powder that make chocolate addictive. Chocolate lovers often admit that they are addicted and find it difficult to resist cravings. When coming down from a chocolate 'high', symptoms include anxiety, migraine, abdominal pain, joint pain, mental agitation and depression. Whilst chocolate addiction is socially acceptable it is still unhealthy – plus, it contributes to obesity.

Sugar

Simple sugars

Sugar is used in all kinds of foods and drinks, in many different forms. However, sugar is, in fact, a harmful substance and contains no nutrients whatsoever, these having been destroyed in the refining process. Worse still, sugar leaches the body of nutrients, and cannot be digested. It causes tooth decay, is a major factor in obesity, it weakens the pancreas and liver, and upsets the levels of glucose in the blood, increasing the risk of diabetes and cardiovascular disease. If that were not enough, it has also been linked to conditions like allergies and degenerative diseases.

Molasses, syrups, dextrose, glucose and fructose are also examples of simple sugars. They do not need digestion and are rapidly absorbed into our bloodstream, causing problems for the body.

Complex sugars

Fruit contains a natural form of sugar called fructose. Fortunately for us, it also contains vitamins, minerals and enzymes, and is an example of a complex carbohydrate (a complete food). The nutrients and co-factors present in this complex carbohydrate are necessary for the body to make use of the glucose.

Sugar and diabetes

In due course, both simple and complex sugars break down into glucose, which is readily absorbed through the digestive tract and goes immediately into the bloodstream.

Glucose is necessary for cell function, especially brain function. The level of glucose in the blood is crucial – too much and the body can become diabetic; too little and we pass out. The body has its own mechanism for balancing blood sugar, with a diet of natural, unprocessed foods.

When sugar is absorbed into the bloodstream, it causes blood glucose levels to rise. Excess consumption of sugar can result in these levels becoming too high – a condition known as hyperglycaemia. If the pancreas functions efficiently, it will produce enough insulin to remove the excess glucose from the bloodstream.

Unfortunately, this huge production of insulin cannot be stopped once it has started. The excess insulin will then cause a rapid fall of glucose levels in the blood – a condition known as hypoglycaemia.

Symptoms can include aggression, depression, dizziness, insomnia, weakness and loss of consciousness. What is more, when blood glucose falls too low, the adrenal glands activate the body's stores of glycogen (a starch-like carbohydrate stored mainly in the liver and muscles) and will also stimulate the synthesis of glucose from proteins and other substances present in the body.

An excess of sugars in the diet overburdens the pancreas and adrenal glands, which weakens them and eventually results in cardiovascular problems and diabetes. If the body cannot use all of the extra fats and cholesterol produced from these sugars, it can be deposited in the cells of the arteries, fat tissues, heart, kidneys, liver, muscles and other organs.

Sugar and the immune system

Sugar suppresses the immune system and increases the body's chances of diseases caused by poor immune function, e.g. allergies, colds, flu, fatigue and infections.

1. Firstly, sugar obstructs the digestion, allowing undigested food into the bloodstream – thereby slowing down the circulation and reducing activity of white blood cells.

2. Secondly, the immune system becomes sensitized to refined sugar. This means that, over time, the immune system adapts to excessive levels of sugar and no longer triggers such a violent response – resulting in a decline of overall health.

Do not replace sugar with artificial sweeteners like saccharin or aspartame as these are also detrimental to your health. Minimize your consumption of sugar in all forms and use natural sweeteners such as raw honey, real maple syrup or Stevia granules, instead.

Stevia (sugar alternative)

Stevia is a natural, low-calorie sweetener with a taste very close to that of cane sugar. Extracted from Stevia leaves it has a high sweetness level (up to 300 times that of cane sugar) yet is extremely low in calories (1/300 that of cane sugar). It is available in powder, granulated, liquid and tablet form. I recommend that only *'Stevia Blend Granulated'* is used for my recipes. Because it is granulated and pre-blended with Erythritol, it is easier to gauge the amount needed for each recipe. If powdered or liquid Stevia were to be used, it would take much trial and error before the correct ratio is found.

Research has revealed that Stevia has no toxic side-effects, is non-carcinogenic and safe for human consumption. If used as an alternative to cane sugar in food and drinks, it can help prevent many common diseases, e.g. high blood pressure, diabetes, obesity, heart disease and tooth decay.

Cancer

Everyone has cancer cells in their body. But these cancer cells don't show up in test results until they have multiplied to a few billion. If the immune system is strong, cancer cells will be destroyed and prevented from multiplying and forming tumours.

When cancer is diagnosed, it suggests that the individual has numerous nutritional deficiencies, possibly due to genetic, environmental, food and lifestyle origins. To overcome these nutritional deficiencies, a change of diet and the inclusion of supplements will strengthen the immune system.

Medical intervention

With conventional treatments (chemotherapy and radiotherapy), the immune system is either compromised or destroyed, leaving the patient open to various kinds of infections and complications.

Chemotherapy and radiotherapy can cause cancer cells to mutate and become resistant to treatment. Surgery can also cause cancer cells to spread to other parts of the body.

However, an effective way to combat cancer is to starve the cancer cells by not feeding them the foods they need to multiply.

What do cancer cells feed on?

Sugar feeds cancer. By eliminating sugar from the diet it cuts off one important food supply to the cancer cells. Sugar substitutes are made with saccharine or aspartame, which are harmful to the body. A better natural alternative would be Manuka honey, Stevia granules or molasses – but only in very small amounts.

Milk causes the body to generate mucus, particularly in the gastro-intestinal tract. Cancer feeds on mucus. By avoiding cow's milk and switching to unsweetened almond milk or soya milk, cancer cells are starved.

Cancer cells flourish in an acidic environment. Red meat is acidic and eating fish and a little chicken is a better option than beef, lamb or pork. Meat also contains livestock antibiotics and growth hormones, which are harmful to a healthy person, even more so to someone with cancer.

Fibre and bowel cancer

Recent research has indicated that eating foods high in fibre can reduce the risk of bowel cancer. Individuals who consumed the most fibre had a 25-40% lower risk of bowel cancer compared to those who ate the least.

It is believed that butyrate, a chemical produce by bacteria and fibre interacting together, changes the conditions in the bowel, so that tumours are less likely to develop. Research has shown that butyrate can also halt the growth of cancer cells and kill them off.

Fruit & vegetables and cancer

Various studies have shown that people who consume plenty of fruit and vegetables can lower their risk of cancer by about a quarter compared to those who eat the bare minimum. In particular, eating lots of fruit and vegetables could reduce the risk of mouth, oesophageal and laryngeal cancers by at least a third, and the risk of lung cancer by at least a quarter.

However, researchers are still unable to say which of the many nutrients in fruit and vegetables are responsible for reducing the risk of cancer. At present, studies are targeting vitamin E, and folate (a naturally occurring form of folic acid).

Nevertheless, it is possible that we need all of these nutrients in balanced combinations to effectively reduce the risk of cancer. Fruit and vegetables of different colours contain different nutrients so it is important to eat as wide range of colours as possible. One study concluded that individuals who consume the widest range of fruit and vegetables have a 22% lower risk of mouth cancer than those who eat the smallest range.

Just as important is the fact that there is strong evidence to suggest that the nutrients found in fruit and vegetables do not reduce the risk of cancer when they are taken in the form of supplements.

Eating the recommended five portions of fruit and vegetables a day can help reduce the risk of bowel, breast, kidney, womb and oesophageal cancers, as well as reducing the risk of other diseases like heart disease and diabetes. A recent study found that people who consumed the most fruit and vegetables reduced their risk of dying from diseases like heart diseases, cancer and diabetes by a quarter.

Red or processed meat and cancer

Various studies have concluded that consuming large amounts of red or processed meat increases the risk of bowel cancer. Red meat includes all fresh, minced and frozen beef, pork and lamb. Processed meat includes ham, bacon, salami and sausages. It was found that eating two daily 80g portions of these meats increases the bowel cancer risk by a third, compared to eating just 20g a day, and that processed meat increases the risk of bowel cancer more than red meat.

There is strong evidence linking red meat to pancreatic and stomach cancer. People consuming in excess of 100g of meat a day had over 3 times the risk of developing stomach cancer. Another extensive study found that those who eat the most red or processed meat have 40-50% higher risk of pancreatic cancer.

Fortunately, there is no strong evidence that eating white meat (such as chicken or turkey) can increase the risk of cancer.

Fish and bowel cancer

Scientists have reported that individuals who eat an 80g portion of fish a day reduce their bowel cancer risk by a third compared to people who eat less than that in a week. Whilst other studies have shown similar results, the evidence is still inconsistent.

Just how eating fish might reduce the risk of cancer is still unknown. We know that fish oils are rich in omega-3 fatty acids but there is no clear evidence that these can reduce the risk of cancer.

Saturated fat and breast cancer

The link between fat and breast cancer is a contentious subject. Scientists disagree over whether the amount of fat we eat affects the risk of breast cancer.

However, two of the largest studies have shown that women who eat the most saturated fat have a higher risk of breast cancer. Fat in our diets probably increases the levels of oestrogen and other hormones in our blood, thereby increasing the risk of breast cancer.

Salt and stomach cancer

There is evidence that eating excessive amounts of salty food, or food that has been preserved with salt, could increase the risk of stomach cancer by damaging the lining of the stomach and causing inflammation. It is also possible that salt interacts with a stomach bug called helicobacter pylori, known to cause both stomach ulcers and stomach cancer.

Helping yourself

To help put the body in an alkaline environment, it is best to adopt a diet made up of 80% fresh vegetables and juice, seeds, nuts, whole grains, and a little fruit (only 20% of this should be from cooked food including beans).

Fresh vegetable juices provide live enzymes that are easily absorbed and reach down to cellular levels within 15 minutes to nourish and enhance growth of healthy cells. To obtain live enzymes for building healthy cells try and drink fresh vegetable juice (most vegetables including bean sprouts) and eat some raw vegetables 2 or 3 times a day. Enzymes are destroyed at temperatures of 40°C).

Do not drink coffee, tea and chocolate (these contain high amounts of caffeine). Green tea is a better option and has cancer-fighting properties. Drink only filtered or purified water as tap water contains toxins and heavy metals. Also avoid distilled water as it is acidic.

Supplements that support the immune system (such as antioxidants, vitamins, minerals etc) facilitate the body to destroy existing cancer cells. Vitamin E is known to cause apoptosis (programmed cell death), the body's natural means of eliminating damaged or unwanted cells.

Cancer cells cannot thrive in an oxygenated atmosphere, so regular exercise and deep breathing will help to get more oxygen down to the cellular level where it can do most good. Oxygen therapy is another means employed to destroy cancer cells.

BENEFICIAL FOODS

Apple cider vinegar

The fermented fruit acid in apple cider vinegar is packed with beneficial vitamins and minerals, including potassium, magnesium, calcium, iron, other trace minerals, and pectin. Pectin is a fibre and it is thought that it can attach itself to cholesterol particles and remove them from the body. It is also believed to help with thinning the blood, improving circulation, and reducing high blood pressure.

Cider vinegar is known traditionally as an excellent detoxifying food, breaking down mucus and phlegm in the body, and for the relief of arthritis as it breaks down the acid crystals that can harden in the joints and cause pain. Research shows that by adding apple cider vinegar to food, calcium absorption is increased.

It also helps to control negative bacteria, so adding three cups of pure apple cider vinegar and a few drops of tea tree essential oil to your bath can be beneficial when you have a vaginal infection.

Coconut oil

Coconut oil contains a high level of saturated fat. But don't panic! Recent research has shown that not all saturated fats are alike. The fatty acids in coconut oil (medium chain triglycerides) do not raise cholesterol or contribute towards heart disease, nor do they promote platelet stickiness or blood clot formation. In fact, they are very healthy. Asian cultures eat significant amounts of coconut in their diet yet do not suffer from many of the diseases prevalent in the west.

The benefits of coconut oil

- Supports a healthy metabolic function and immune system
- Is a protective antioxidant
- Helps control diabetes
- Helps keep the skin soft and smooth and protect against skin cancer and other blemishes
- Helps prevent bacterial, viral, and fungal infections
- Helps prevent osteoporosis
- Improves digestion and the absorption of nutrients
- Promotes weight loss and is lower in calories than other fats
- Reduces the risk of atherosclerosis and related illnesses
- Reduces the risk of cancer and other degenerative conditions
- Supplies important nutrients essential for good health and is an immediate source of energy.

Superfoods

We all need vitamins and minerals – however, research has uncovered an abundance of phytonutrients (from phytochemicals) that have acknowledged benefits to health not provided by vitamins or minerals. Phytochemicals are chemical compounds such as beta-carotene that occur naturally in plants and foods containing these phytochemicals are called Superfoods.

Including Superfoods in our daily diet is the simplest way to get the widest variety of these compounds. In fact, an abundance of phytonutrients, along with live enzymes, essential fats, vitamins and minerals, metabolites, and many other health-giving compounds are to be found in a single Superfood.

It goes without saying that the wider the variety of Superfoods we consume, the wider our intake of phytonutrients and other nutritional compounds, the health benefits of which may include increased energy; strengthened immunity; support of the bones, joints and cardiovascular system; improved skin, hair and nails; etc.

Superfoods also contain compounds that may boost the efficacy of vitamins and minerals within supplements.

Below is a list of easily obtainable Superfoods. Remember to vary your daily intake for optimal health:

- Almonds
- Apples
- Avocados
- Baked beans
- Bananas
- Beetroot
- Blueberries
- Brazil nuts
- Broccoli
- Ginger
- Green tea
- Olive oil
- Onions
- Oranges
- Pumpkins
- Salmon
- Soya
- Spirulina powder
- Cocoa (organic)
- Cranberries
- Flaxseed
- Garlic
- Tomatoes
- Whole grains
- Yogurt (live).

Hot flushes eased with flaxseed

The inclusion of flaxseed in your daily diet could help to reduce hot flushes – a common symptom of oestrogen deficiency experienced during the menopause. Whilst the plant soya has been shown to help reduce the symptoms of menopause, further study suggests that flaxseed is another phytoestrogen that works equally well. Flaxseed also contains Omega 3, making it doubly beneficial to the body. Why not try it for yourself by adding flaxseed oil to salads or sprinkle a few seeds over salads or snacks.

Herbs to help lower your blood pressure

Lowering blood pressure with the aid of herbs is an acknowledged alternative to diuretics, a practice that has been carried out in countries like India and some parts of Asia for many years.

Garlic

One natural high blood pressure treatment, proven to keep cholesterol and heart related problems away, is garlic. Research has found that it inhibits clot formation by making platelets less likely to clump together, thus avoiding artery-clogging plaques. The recommended daily amount for a person with high blood pressure is one to two cloves.

Indian ginseng

Ashwagandha (Indian Ginseng) is another herb proven to bring good results for blood pressure. It has properties that help the body adapt to and cope with a variety of stresses. In the elderly, it is best taken with almond milk to tackle insomnia brought on by stress and hypertension. Take a daily dose of 3-6g of the root powder with lukewarm water.

Indian pennywort

Gotu Kola (Indian pennywort) has also been confirmed as a wonderful herb for blood pressure and is best known for its tranquillity enhancing property. This herb has been used for hypertensive patients to relax them, cleanse the blood, and increase function of the brain. Prepare the pennywort by boiling it in water and take 20-30 ml, diluted in equal water, twice daily. In powder form, take 3-6g per day with lukewarm water.

Aloe vera

Aloe vera is yet another herb commonly used to lower blood pressure. The glycoproteins and polysaccharides it contains are believed to be beneficial for many illnesses. Glycoproteins trigger rapid healing and halt pain and inflammation; while polysaccharides promote skin growth and repair. Both elements also help to control blood sugar levels – hence, a good cure for diabetes. Take 20 ml of Aloe vera juice twice daily, diluted with equal water.

Hawthorn

Hawthorn can be safely consumed by persons with high blood pressure who are already taking medications. Research has shown that taking this herb can have optimal effect in just four weeks. Hawthorn is said to dilate coronary blood vessels. Take between 160-900 mg of hawthorn leaf and flower daily for six weeks.

Coleus forskohlii

Another herb, which is used in Ayurvedic medicine, is Coleus forskohlii. Research has proven it to have hypertensive and antispasmodic effects. Its blood pressure lowering effects appear to be due to relaxation of the arterial vascular smooth muscle.

OVERVIEW

- Do not use sugar or flour
- Do not eat processed foods or red meat
- Do not eat meat or fish if you have been diagnosed with cancer. However, when it has been overcome, then you may eat a small amount of organic meat and fish but red meat should **never** be eaten
- Do not use dairy foods apart from the one breakfast recipe I mentioned of cottage cheese and flaxseed oil
- Avoid stimulants i.e. coffee, tea, carbonated drinks, alcohol and chocolate
- Eat nuts and seeds (almonds, apricot kernels – not more than 2-3 per day)
- Avoid fizzy drinks and any other sweet artificially made refreshment
- See a Medical Herbalist to prescribe herbs suitable for your specific need

- Eat raw vegetables and a little fruit on a daily basis; these should be organic or alternatively, try growing your own, if possible (see **How to Grow Your Own Produce** on page 157)

- Eat beans, pulses and seeds, lentils and mung beans, quinoa, sesame seeds, linseeds and more

- Use coconut oil as a nutritional alternative to traditional oils

- Use spices such as ginger to aid sickness, turmeric powder for its anti-cancer properties, garlic and more

- Do not cook your food on high heat

- Drink green tea for its antioxidant properties and drink plenty of purified water.

BREAKFAST

Never miss breakfast

Eating breakfast is essential for optimal health. Not only does it help in balancing blood sugar levels, but research has shown that omitting this vital meal from your daily diet can raise cholesterol levels. Skipping breakfast was linked to a considerably higher total LDL cholesterol level and increased insulin sensitivity, both of which could lead to weight gain over time.

Riki's muesli

Ingredients:

¼ cup soaked pumpkin seeds

½ cup soaked almonds

1 tbsp dried coconut flakes

¼ cup pine seeds

½ cup almond or walnut milk

¼ cup mulberry fruit or goji berries

½ cup fresh blueberry, raspberries (if in season) otherwise try apple & banana

Preparation:

- Blend the pumpkin seeds, almonds, coconut and pine seeds for a moment or two until slightly coarse.
- Add the mulberry fruit or goji berries and mix together.
- Place in glass jar with a seal and place in the fridge (this mix can be kept for 2 days only, then make a new batch).
- Serve with fresh blueberries, raspberries or apple and banana, add the almond milk and enjoy!

EASY

Nutrition:

Great source of dietary fibre, antioxidant, essential fatty acids, calcium and potassium.

Porridge

(see picture on page 47)

Ingredients:

3-4 tbsp organic medium oatmeal

Almond milk or water

½ tsp cinnamon

½ fresh green apple cut into small cubes

1 tsp Manuka honey

Preparation:

- Put the oatmeal and the almond milk or water in a saucepan and stir together.
- Heat on a low heat with some of the cinnamon.
- As soon as you see the mix begin to boil, remove and place in a breakfast dish.
- Add the apple, honey and cinnamon and enjoy.

You can also eat your porridge with blueberries and/or goji berries to sweeten it and raise your energy.

EASY

Nutrition:

A bowl of hot porridge is especially warming on cold winter mornings. It is best to use steel-cut oats (whole oat groats, cut into small pieces). They are more nutritious than rolled or quick oats, which, due to processing, are lacking in some nutrients.

Whole oats contain soluble fibre, selenium, thiamin, phosphorus and manganese, as well as small amounts of copper, folic acid, vitamin E, and zinc. If you are on a gluten-free diet, try using millet or quinoa. Millet is more substantial, while quinoa is much lighter and fluffier than most whole grains.

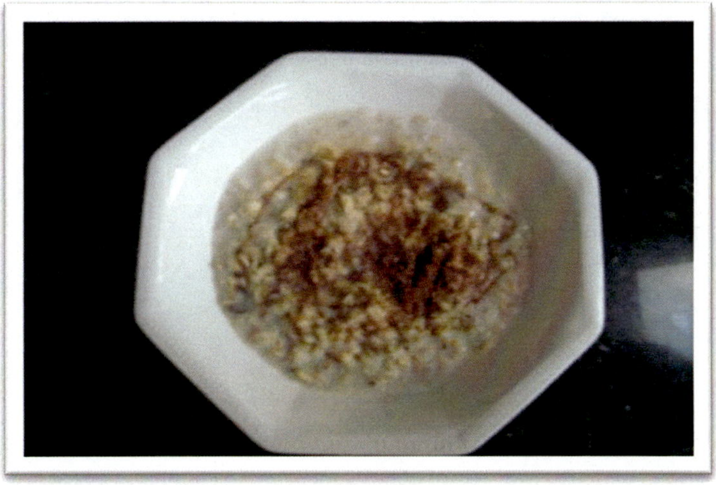

Porridge

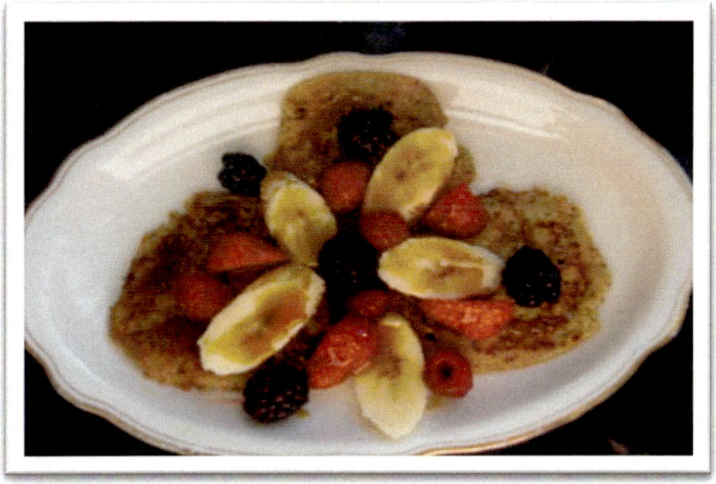

Nutritious & tasty pancake

Cottage cheese/flaxseed oil mix

Ingredients:

1/3 cup flaxseed oil

2/3 cup cottage cheese

Mixed berries

1 apple

Juice of ½ pomegranate

10 almonds

2 walnuts

Preparation:

- Mix the flaxseed oil and the cottage cheese thoroughly in a bowl (the oil will not be noticeable once it has bonded with the cheese).
- Place the mix in a blender and add the rest of the ingredients; blend for a few seconds.
- Add a little water, if necessary.

EASY

Nutrition:

Although cottage cheese is a dairy product, when mixed thoroughly with flaxseed oil it loses its dairy properties. This dish is low in calories, cholesterol and sodium, full of antioxidants, vitamin C, and potassium and is a good source of protein and fibre.

Nutritious & tasty pancake

(see picture on page 47)

Ingredients:

1 cup of fine oat flour

1 cup organic barley flour

Pinch of Celtic sea salt

1 cup almond milk

1 organic egg

Coconut oil or olive oil (for the pan)

Manuka honey or yacon syrup

Mixture of fresh, seasonal fruit (optional)

Preparation:

- Mix together the oats, barley flour, salt, almond milk, and egg.
- Heat one spoonful of either olive or coconut oil in a pan. Add some of the pancake mix and let it cook.
- When ready, put on a plate and add syrup to taste and fruit (if desired).

EASY

Nutrition:

Oat has a soluble fibre beta-glucans known to reduce blood cholesterol. It is a source of calcium, potassium and energy.

Make your own almond milk

(see picture on page 52)

Almond milk is an excellent substitute for cow's milk. However, not all commercially prepared almond milks are suitable. Anyone watching their blood sugar and insulin levels would have problems with the added sugar in some brands, whilst others have added synthetic vitamins and minerals to make it resemble cow's milk when comparing nutrition. Fortunately, you can make your own natural almond milk quite simply and cheaply.

Ingredients:

1 to 1½ cups almonds

4 cups water

3-8 dates (optional)

Preparation:

- Soak almonds in water for at least 8 hours.
- Drain soaked almonds, and blend with 4 cups of fresh water until you get a milk-like consistency.
- Blend with dates that have been soaked for at least an hour (optional for sweetness).
- Sieve the milk through a muslin cloth and squeeze it all out until you get pure milk.

This all-natural almond milk keeps for four to five days in an air-tight jar in the refrigerator.

MODERATELY EASY

Nutrition:

This delicious, creamy milk is free from added oils, concentrated sugars and synthetic nutrients.

Variations

Alternatively, you can make seed milk, substituting the nuts for hemp, sunflower, sesame or pumpkin seeds. Each has its own individual flavour, so try them to see which you like best both as a drink and as a base for smoothies and shakes. Almond milk is a staple among raw food fans as it has a delicate taste that complements any flavour you add to it. The milk can be as watery or as creamy as you like by changing the proportion of nuts to liquid. It is even possible to make whipped cream by blending soaked cashews or macadamias with an equal volume of water.

Getting organized

Why not blend up a big batch of your favourite raw milk every few days and keep it in a sealed container in your fridge? That way you will always have it to hand whenever you fancy a nutritious drink, or need some as a base for a recipe.

Shakes and smoothies

Nut and seed milks make an excellent base for shakes and smoothies of all kinds. You can add flavourings such as coconut butter, vanilla, carob or mesquite powder, and you can blend them with fruits, and/or with a mix of superfoods such as maca, blue-green algae, tocotrienols (a rich source of natural vitamin E) or any high-quality powdered green supplement.

The benefits of almonds

Anyone dedicated to a healthy lifestyle should always include nutritious almonds in their daily diet. Almonds are cholesterol free, low in saturated fat, and high in protein. They contain vitamins A and E, thiamin, riboflavin, niacin, vitamin B6, folic acid, vitamin B12, pantothenic acid, biotin, vitamins C and D, sodium, potassium, iron, calcium, magnesium, phosphorous, zinc, copper and healthy fibre. They also have anti-cancer and anti-inflammatory properties, and help build a healthy heart.

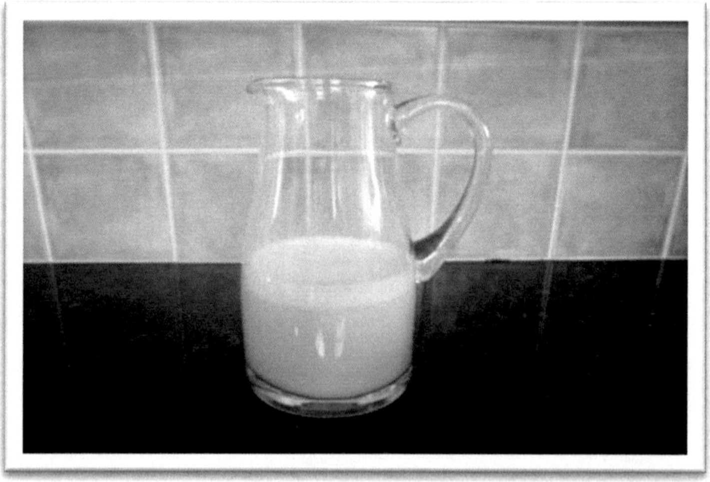

Almond milk

SMOOTHIES

Mixed nuts & banana milkshake

Ingredients:

1 banana

½ cup mixed nuts (almonds, walnuts, brazil nuts)

½ cup water

Ice

Preparation:

- Soak the mixed nuts in water for 2 hours prior to making the shake
- Put this mix in a blender with ½ cup of water and blend
- Sieve the milk through a muslin cloth and squeeze it all out until you get pure milk
- Put the banana in the blender, add the nut milk and ice and blend for 30 seconds and serve this delicious, nutritious milkshake.

MODERATELY EASY

Nutrition:

Good source of dietary fibre, vitamins A, C and B, calcium, iron, potassium, and manganese. Low in saturated fat.

Healthy & refreshing smoothie

Ingredients:

½ apple

3 slices pineapple

1 tsp hemp seeds

¾ cup almond milk

20g freshly sliced coconut

¼ tsp cinnamon

Preparation:

- Grind the hemp seeds using a pestle and mortar.
- Put all the other ingredients into a blender and add the ground hemp seeds and cinnamon – blend and enjoy!

EASY

Nutrition:

Good source of dietary fibre, vitamins A and C, and iron; low in saturated fat and calories. This smoothie has antioxidant properties.

Pineapple helps the body digest food by breaking down protein; it promotes energy and contains essential fatty acids.

Mango delight smoothie

Ingredients:

1 tsp crushed linseeds

½ mango

½ apple

½ cup coconut milk

Ice cubes

Preparation:

- Put all the ingredients in a blender and blend on high speed for 1 minute.
- Pour into a long glass and enjoy!

EASY

Nutrition:

Good source of fibre, vitamins A and C, pectin, and essential fatty acids.

Green smoothie

(see picture on page 58)

Ingredients:

1 banana

¼ cup almond milk

1 tsp green superfood powder

Preparation:

- Blend the banana along with the green super food powder and almond milk.
- Pour into a long glass.

EASY

Nutrition:

Contains a wide variety of minerals, vitamins and cancer-fighting phytonutrients.

This smoothie is very appealing colour-wise to young children as well as adults and is very nutritious.

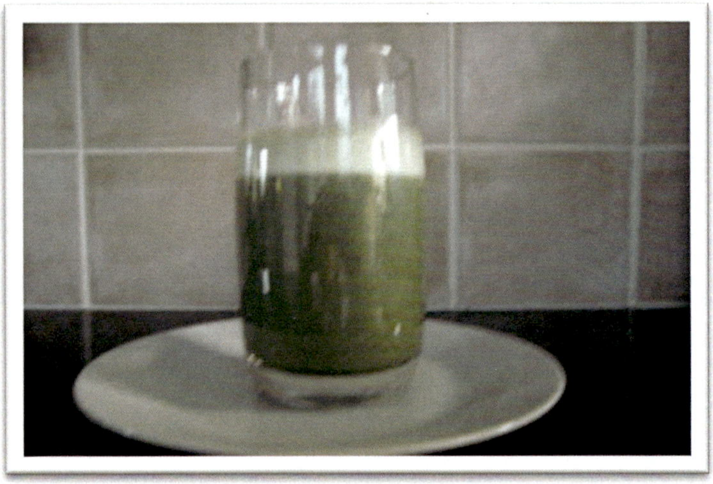

Green smoothie

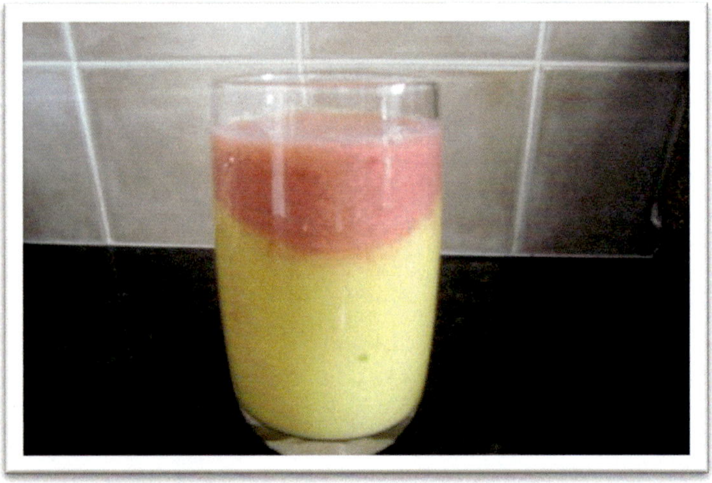

Mango & strawberry shake

Mango & strawberry shake

(see picture on page 58)

Ingredients:

½ mango	½ cup almond milk
10 strawberries	Ice cubes

Preparation:

- Blend the mango with half of the almond milk and some ice then pour into a glass.
- Blend the strawberries with the remaining almond milk and ice cubes and gently pour over the mango by dribbling it over the back of a spoon.

You can also mix strawberries and blueberries to make it dark red on top of the mango. Very appetising and appealing to children!

EASY

Nutrition:

A good source of vitamins A, C, and B6, calcium and iron, folic acid and potassium. Strawberry is a heart-friendly fruit and helps reduce blood pressure.

JUICES

Drinking just one glass of freshly made vegetable juice a day is a simple and refreshing way of treating your body to a host of vitamins, minerals and phytonutrients. Whilst being highly nutritional, it benefits the human body by protecting cells against disease and premature ageing.

Practically any vegetables are suitable for juicing but be wary of using too many carrots, sweet root vegetables and fruit, which need to be added in small quantities. Although they are undoubtedly healthy, they should never make up more than one-third of the whole drink.

Organic vegetables are free from harmful chemicals and have the benefit of being much tastier than non-organic, so why not take a look at the chapter on **How to Grow your Own Produce** on page 105 and attempt to grow your own? It's so rewarding – you'll be glad you gave it a go!

(Please refer to **Useful Links** on page 197 for information on good juicers.)

Cleanse your body and strengthen your immune system

10g ginger

1 carrot

½ apple

Cleanse your skin and improve bad breath

½ apple

1 carrot

1 tomato

Eliminate toxins, aid high blood pressure and headache and water retention

2 celery stalks

1 apple

1 small size cucumber

Revive and energise the kidneys and bladder

½ apple

2 slices watermelon

2 pineapple rings

Cleanse and improve skin

1 kiwi

2 celery stalks

1 apple

Body warming and digestive stimulant

1 carrot

10g ginger

2 pineapple rings

Source of vitamin C and to relieve constipation

1 banana

1 pear

1 papaya

10 grapes

Cleansing and refreshing

Handful spinach leaves

1 small cucumber

1 carrot

Digestive stimulant

Handful of spinach

½ fennel bulb

10g ginger

1 garlic clove

1 small cucumber

Blood cleanser

5 leaves of kale

2 carrots

¼ lime

2 celery stalks

Refreshing and full of vitamin C to aid your immune system

10 strawberries

Good slice watermelon

1 banana

Immune system support and skin cleanser

30ml wheatgrass every day

Wheatgrass is the name for the young green shoots of a wheat plant (*Triticum aestium*) and is full of essential vitamins, minerals and amino acids that the human body needs in order to function properly.

Just one tiny 30ml measure of juiced wheatgrass is nutritionally equivalent to around a kilo of leafy green vegetables.

Wheatgrass consists of 70% chlorophyll, which is used by plants to convert sunlight into energy – so get juicing and feel the benefits of this amazing plant!

Pomegranate juice

Good for bad breath and believed to help certain breast cancers by preventing and slowing their growth. A recent study in America has shown that a group of phytochemicals called ellagitannins, which are plentiful in pomegranates, inhibited the growth of oestrogen-responsive breast cancer in laboratory tests.

Pomegranates contain iron, calcium, potassium, magnesium, vitamin C, phosphorus and some vitamin A.

For best results you should juice the whole fruit, including the peel, in a good quality juicer.

LUNCH/DINNER

Riki's majdara

(see picture on page 70)

Ingredients:

150g green lentils

50g barley grain

50g spelt grain

50g brown rice

10-20g fresh ginger

3 garlic cloves

½ tsp rosemary

½ tsp asafoetida yellow powder

½ pint of water

¼ red cabbage

50g seaweed

Rocket

1 beetroot

1 avocado

1 red onion

Dressing:

3 tbsp apple cider vinegar

3 tbsp olive oil or flax oil

½ tsp mustard paste

Very small pinch sea salt, optional

Black pepper

1 tin sardines (optional)

Preparation:

- Place the lentils, barley grain, spelt grain, brown rice, fresh ginger, garlic cloves (unpeeled), rosemary and asafoetida yellow powder in a pan with the water and put on low heat to cook for 20 minutes. When cooked, put aside.

Prepare the dressing:

- Put the sliced red cabbage, seaweed, rocket, grated beetroot, avocado (cut into small cubes) and red onion in a large bowl.

- Add the apple cider, olive or flaxseed oil, mustard, black pepper and a very small pinch of salt to the bowl.
- Then add the contents of the pan and the sardines for essential fatty acid (if required). Mix all together.

MODERATELY EASY

Nutrition:

Do not use barley if you are sensitive to gluten. Seaweed contains vitamins A, B1, B2, B6, C, niacin, iodine, iron, zinc calcium, sodium, potassium, magnesium and a trace of B12.

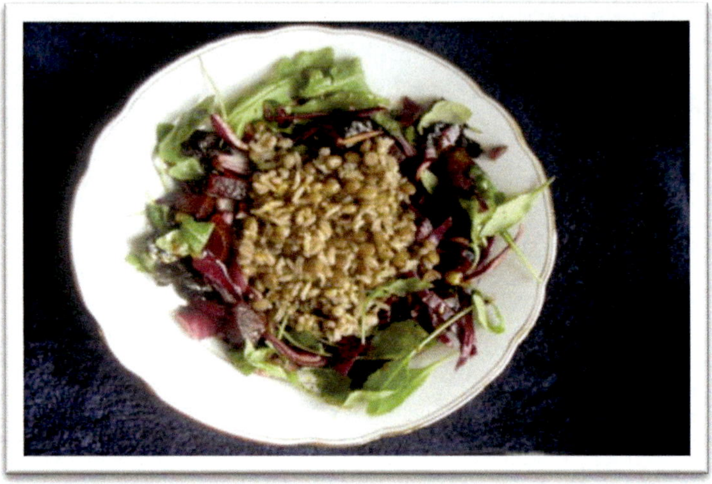

Riki's majdara

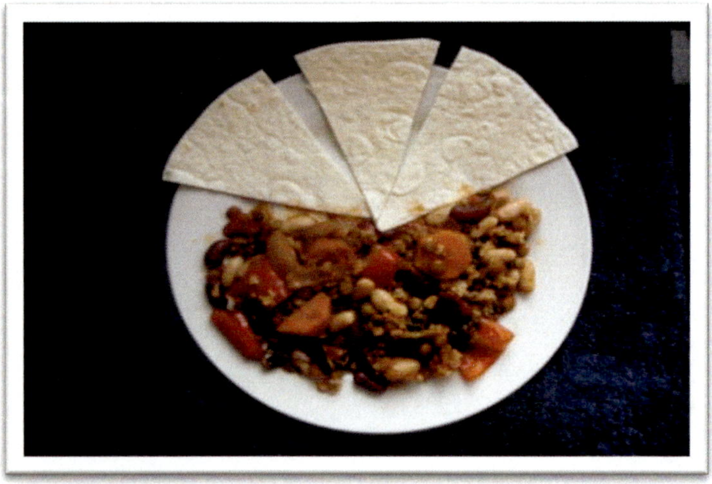

Fresh delicious chilli

Fresh delicious chilli

(see picture on page 70)

Ingredients:

½ cup broad beans
½ cup kidney beans
½ cup green lentils
½ cup organic brown rice
2 large tomatoes
1 large red onion
3-6 cloves garlic
1 fresh red pepper

2 large carrots
2 tsp chilli powder
1 tsp ground cumin
A little grated nutmeg
¼ tsp cayenne pepper
3 bay leaves
Handful fresh coriander

2 tbsp tomato paste
Vegetable or sea salt (optional)
Pinch ground black pepper
1-2 cubes of vegetable stock
Water
2-3 tbsp olive oil

Preparation:

- Soak the broad beans and kidney beans in water for 8 hours or overnight.
- Chop the onion, garlic, carrots and red pepper and place in a saucepan with a little olive oil and cook for 3 minutes.
- Add the spices and tomato paste and mix together while still cooking.

- Put the vegetable stock in a cup, dissolve in hot water then add to the saucepan.
- Add the beans, lentils, rice, bay leaves, coriander leaves, and chopped tomatoes and leave to cook for a further 20-30 minutes on a low heat, adding water as you go along and when needed. Then let it simmer for 5-10 minutes.

This dish can be served with either wholemeal pitta bread or, if you wish to avoid wheat, a bowl of salad and balsamic vinegar. Any leftovers can be kept in the freezer.

MODERATELY EASY

Nutrition:

Low in cholesterol and sodium, a good source of selenium and manganese. Contains vitamins A, C, B6, E and K, calcium, iron, folic acid, magnesium, potassium and zinc. Good source of fibre. Nutmeg is an antioxidant, rich in B-complex, including riboflavin and niacin.

Falafel

(see picture on page 75)

Ingredients:

737g soaked broad beans

297g soaked chickpeas

2 bunches parsley

2 bunches coriander

3 cloves of garlic

1 pod hot green pepper

453g chopped red onions

2 tbsp vegetable salt

½ tsp black pepper

6 tbsp organic fine oatmeal flour

Extra virgin olive oil for frying

Preparation:

- Put the broad beans, chickpeas, parsley, coriander, garlic, hot green pepper and chopped red onion into a blender and blend.
- Empty the contents into a large bowl and add vegetable salt, black pepper and flour and leave to rest for couple of hours.
- Use this mix to make small balls and fry in deep hot oil for a short while until browned. Alternatively, use only half the mix and put the remainder in the freezer for another time.

Falafel can be eaten hot or cold in pitta bread with humus/tahini spread and salad, or on its own.

EASY

Nutrition:

Good source of dietary fibre, rich in protein, manganese, folic acid, calcium, vitamins A, B6, E, K, and zinc. A healthy source of carbohydrates and low in fat.

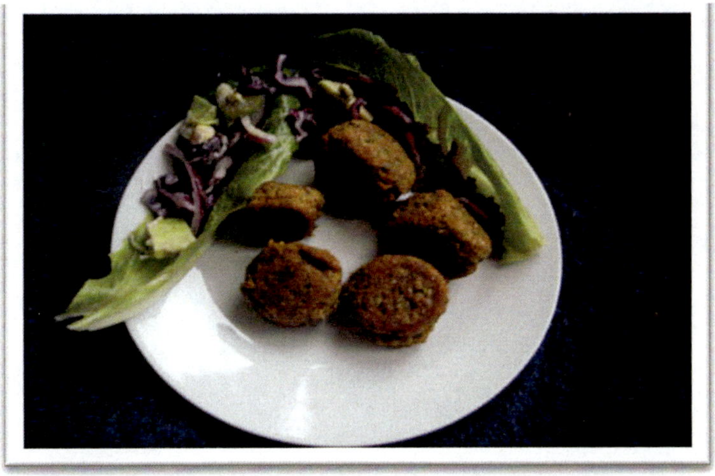

Falafel

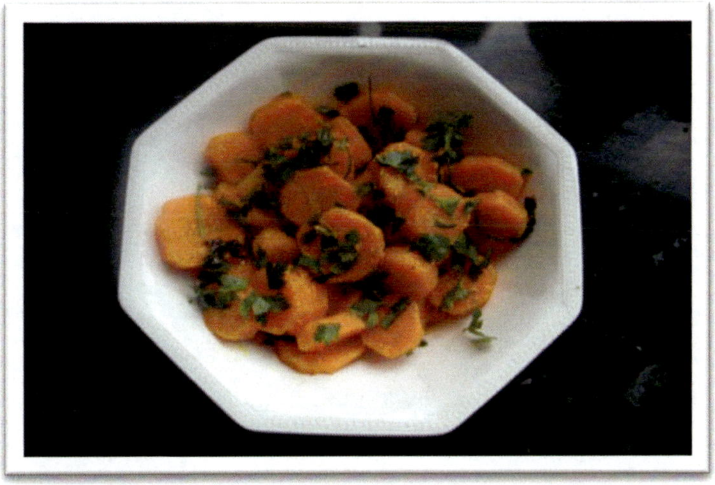

Riki's carrot dish

Stuffed raw red pepper

Ingredients:

2 fresh red peppers

½ cup sunflower seeds

¼ cup pumpkin seeds

¼ cup fenugreek seeds

¼ cup aduki beans

1 small red onion

2 tbsp fresh cashew nut paste

½ cup chopped celery

¼ fresh red chilli

Chopped coriander

Vegetable or Celtic sea salt to taste

Water

Tuna or sardines (optional)

Preparation:

- Put fenugreek seeds and aduki beans in water overnight to soften. Also soak sunflower, pumpkin and cashew nuts in water for 8 hours prior to preparation.
- Sieve the seeds, place in a blender and add water little by little until a paste is formed.
- Add the red chilli, coriander, red onion and salt to taste.
- Cut off the top of the red peppers and empty any seeds from inside.
- You can now stuff the peppers with the paste.
- Alternatively, you can add the tuna or sardines into the paste and then stuff the peppers. Enjoy!

MODERATELY EASY

Nutrition:

This dish is low in saturated fat, sodium and cholesterol. It contains vitamins A, C, E, B5, B6, and K, thiamin, niacin, iron, potassium, folic acid and selenium

It has anti-inflammatory and cardiovascular benefits, contains antioxidants and is a good source of protein, copper, manganese, zinc and essential fatty acids.

Riki's carrot dish

(see picture on page 75)

Ingredients:

4 carrots

Fresh parsley

3 tbsp olive oil

Cumin seeds

Celtic sea salt

Black pepper

½ tsp turmeric

Juice of 1 fresh lemon

Water

Preparation:

- Peel the carrots and cut into 5 mm slices. Place in a saucepan, cover with water, bring to the boil and cook for 15 minutes.
- Leave to cool then put the carrots in a dish and add the olive oil, salt, pepper, cumin seeds, turmeric, and lemon. Mix together and top with some chopped fresh parsley and serve cold or warm.

EASY

Nutrition:

This dish is fat free, cholesterol free and low sodium. It is rich in antioxidants, vitamins (especially vitamins A, B6 and C), calcium, iron, magnesium, and manganese.

Poached fish in vegetables

Ingredients:

Mackerel/salmon/halibut/trout/tuna or sardines

1 carrot

1 green pepper

1 red pepper

3-4 lettuce leaves

2 fresh tomatoes

½ fresh red chilli

½ fresh lemon

Olive oil

2 cloves garlic

½ tsp dried thyme (or one tsp fresh, if available)

½ tsp turmeric powder

Pinch of Celtic sea salt

Preparation:

- Chop all the vegetables into finger size pieces and leave aside.
- Pour the olive oil into a deep pan and, when slightly warm, add the garlic, carrot, green pepper, red pepper and tomatoes and leave to cook for one minute.
- Now add one type of fish as suggested above, the thyme, turmeric powder and a pinch of sea salt and leave to cook for a further 3-4 minutes on a low heat (you can add more water if needed).
- When ready, spread the lettuce on a flat plate and place the vegetables on the lettuce, then the fish on top of the vegetables and garnish with very thin slices of red chilli and the juice of ½ a fresh lemon.

This dish can be served with quinoa, cooked as you would cook rice.

EASY

Nutrition:

Contains essential fatty acids. This dish is low in saturated fat, cholesterol and sodium; contains thiamin, niacin, folic acid, magnesium and copper; is a good source of dietary fibre, vitamins A, C, K, B6 and potassium; has antibacterial, antiviral properties and helps lower risk of cancer.

Nutritious stuffed butternut squash

(see picture on page 83)

Ingredients:

1 butternut squash

1 tsp rosemary (preferably fresh but ¼ tsp of dried can be used)

2 tbsp olive oil

Pinch of salt

Pinch of grated nutmeg

Pinch of black pepper

3 garlic cloves

¼ small fresh chilli

Handful fresh coriander

100g green lentils

50g barley (but do not use if you have a sensitivity to gluten)

50g brown rice

Preparation:

- Place the lentils, barley and brown rice in a saucepan and bring to the boil. Leave aside to cool.
- Preheat the oven to Gas mark 6 or 200°C.
- Halve the butternut, spoon the seeds out and place on a roasting tray.
- Place the rosemary, fresh chilli, garlic, coriander, lentils, barley, rice, olive oil and seasoning in a large bowl and mix together.
- Stuff the butternut with this mix and cook in the oven for 10-15 minutes.

This dish can be eaten with green side salad.

If you made extra filling mix, you can store it in the freezer for next time.

MODERATELY EASY

Nutrition:

Good source of dietary fibre, carbohydrates and protein. Low in fat and high in essential fatty acids. A heart-friendly dish to lower cholesterol due to capsaicin in chilli.

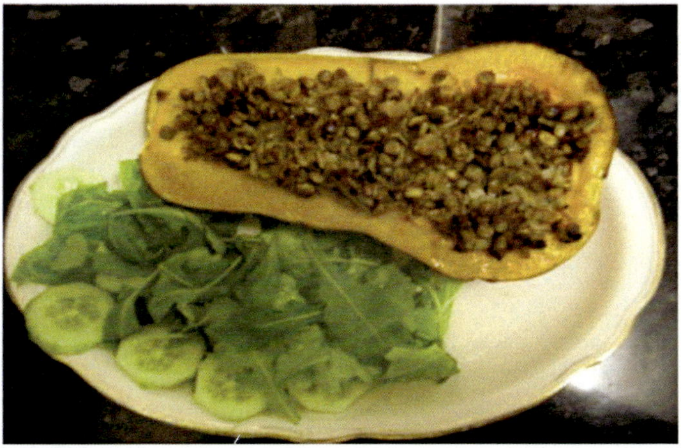

Nutritious stuffed butternut squash

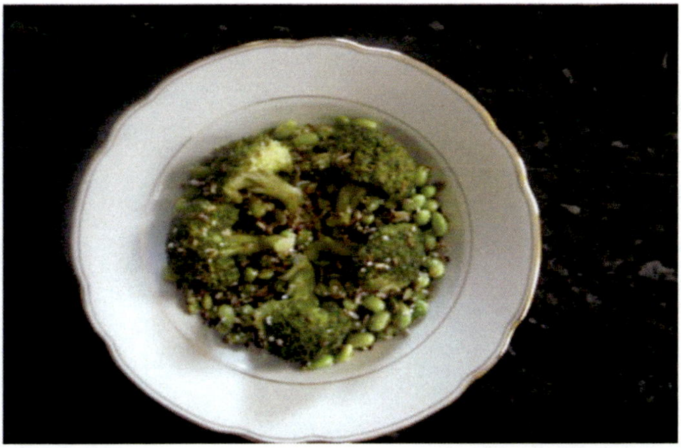

Steamed green beans & broccoli

Steamed green beans & broccoli

(see picture on page 83)

Ingredients:

Small pack of fresh green beans	1 tbsp sunflower seeds
One head of broccoli	1 tsp sesame seeds
2 tbsp olive oil	1 fresh clove garlic
Apple balsamic vinegar	Black pepper to taste

Preparation:

- Cut the broccoli and prepare the green beans, leaving them full length. Place in the steamer and cook for 5-10 minutes.
- When ready place on a plate, add the olive oil, apple balsamic vinegar, sunflower seeds, black pepper and sesame seeds and serve with your chosen meal.

EASY

Nutrition:

This dish is low in calories and contains no saturated fat. It is a good source of essential fatty acids, fibre, vitamin A, antioxidants and beta-carotene, B6, B1, C, iron, magnesium, calcium, potassium and manganese.

Sweet potato dish

(see picture on page 87)

Ingredients:

2 medium sweet potatoes, washed and unpeeled

½ cup cashew nuts

2 tbsp extra-virgin olive oil

2 tbsp fresh lemon juice

Pinch of sea salt

Small amount of fresh coriander

1/3 red cabbage

1 large onion

½ tsp turmeric

Pinch of black pepper

Preparation:

- You can either steam the sweet potatoes (as I prefer) or place them in a saucepan with water and cook for 15 minutes until soft.
- While the sweet potatoes are cooking, cut the cabbage and onion into slices and very quickly stir-fry the onion and cabbage in 2 tbsp olive oil; add the cashew nuts and season with salt, pepper and turmeric.
- Drain the water from the potatoes and let them cool for a short while; then cut into 2.5 cm slices.
- Put the sliced potatoes on a dish and add the stir-fried mix on top, add the lemon juice and garnish with some chopped fresh coriander. Enjoy!

MODERATELY EASY

Nutrition:

Sweet potatoes are a good source of vitamin C and beta-carotene, and are rich in copper, dietary fibre, iron, manganese, potassium and vitamin B6.

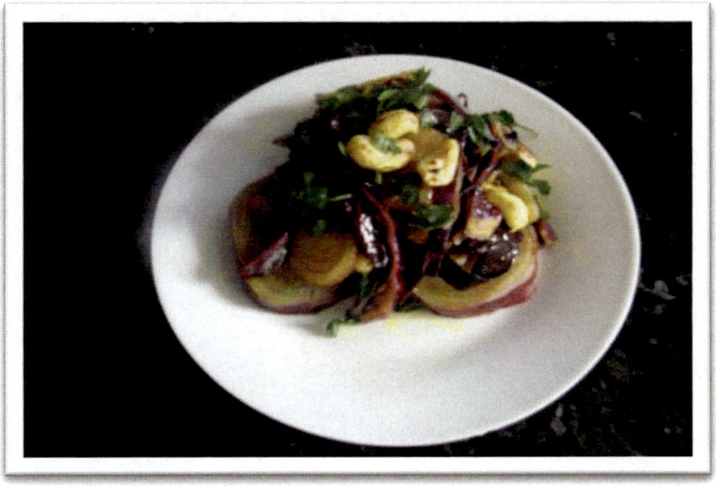

Sweet potato dish

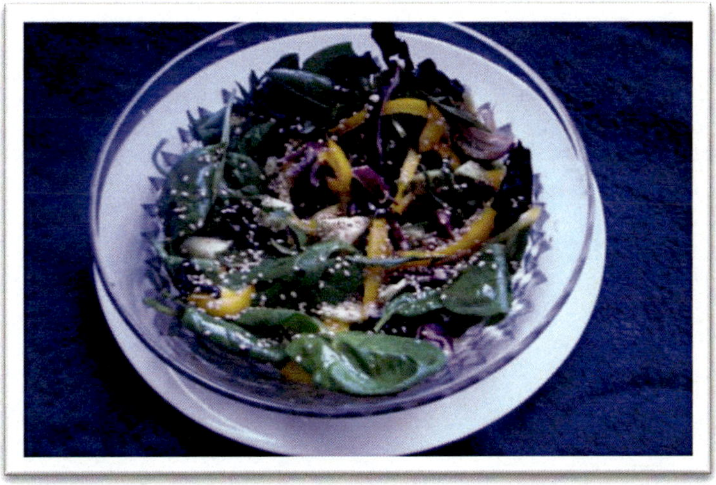

Cabbage & dulse salad

Roasted Jerusalem artichoke bulb (root)

This is a very special dish and not easy to find readily available. Try growing Jerusalem artichokes in your garden and when the yellow flower is dying down, pull the stalk to reveal the root. You'll be surprised when you see the size of the bulb that mimics a sweet potato.

Ingredients:

1-2 bulbs Jerusalem artichoke

Olive oil

Pinch of Celtic sea salt

Black pepper

Fresh lemon juice

Baking foil

Preparation:

- Wash the bulbs, wrap in baking foil and place in the oven for 10-15 minutes on 180-200°C.
- When baked, place on the plate and add the olive oil, pinch of Celtic sea salt and pepper (if required) and a squeeze of fresh lemon juice.

You can also use Jerusalem artichokes in vegetable soup.

EASY

Nutrition:

Jerusalem artichoke is a great vegetable to reduce fat and control the Glycaemic Index, which is of benefit to those with diabetes. It also acts as a pro-biotic due to its insulin content, and is a good source of potassium, iron, calcium, magnesium, copper, selenium, protein, vitamin C and some vitamin B.

Tasty & easy avocado salad

Ingredients:

2 tomatoes

1 good sized avocado

1 small cucumber

Olive oil

Lemon juice or balsamic vinegar to taste

Preparation:

- Chop the tomatoes, avocado and cucumber into small pieces.
- Add the olive oil and lemon juice or balsamic vinegar and enjoy this fresh and nutritious salad.

EASY

Nutrition:

Avocado is high in monounsaturated fatty acids. It is a good source of potassium, iron, copper, phosphorus, magnesium, and dietary fibre, and contains vitamins A, B3, B-complex, C, E and calcium. It helps to control the Glycaemic Index, which is of benefit to those with diabetes.

Cabbage & dulse salad

(see picture on page 87)

Ingredients:

½ small red cabbage

2 tbsp dulse sea vegetable

Handful of spinach

1 yellow pepper

1 avocado

2 tbsp flaxseed oil

2 tbsp balsamic vinegar

½ red onion (optional)

2 tbsp sesame seeds

Handful of chopped fresh coriander

Handful of rocket

Celtic sea salt (if necessary but not recommended)

Preparation:

- Put the dulse in a small bowl with cold water and leave for 1-2 minutes.
- Shred all the vegetables into small pieces and place in a salad bowl.
- Add the oil, balsamic vinegar and a dash of salt and mix together.
- Arrange the mixture on a salad dish.
- Sieve the dulse and put on top of the salad.
- Sprinkle the sesame seeds on top, and this colourful, nutritional salad is ready to serve.

EASY

Nutrition:

This dish is very high in dietary fibre, calcium, manganese, potassium, vitamins B5, B6, C, with a small amount of carbohydrate, protein and beta-carotene. It is a great source of vitamin K, and contains no cholesterol or fat. It is high in essential fatty acids, magnesium, thiamin and iron.

Cabbage and dulse contain sodium, so adding salt is not recommended.

Side salad

(see picture on page 94)

Ingredients:

¼ red cabbage

1 cucumber

10g fresh ginger

½ cup shredded celeriac

Juice of ½ lime

¼ tbsp balsamic vinegar

Celtic sea salt to taste

Black pepper to taste

1 tbsp olive oil

Preparation:

- Cut the red cabbage and cucumber into thin slices and place in a bowl, add the shredded ginger and celeriac.
- Combine the lime juice, balsamic vinegar, salt, pepper and olive oil, add to the salad, mix and serve alongside your chosen dish.

EASY

Nutrition:

This is a good source of dietary fibre. It has no saturated fat or cholesterol. Contains potassium, antioxidants (e.g. beta-carotene, vitamins C and A), and good amounts of vitamins K, B6, magnesium and manganese. It is also a digestive aid due to the health properties of ginger.

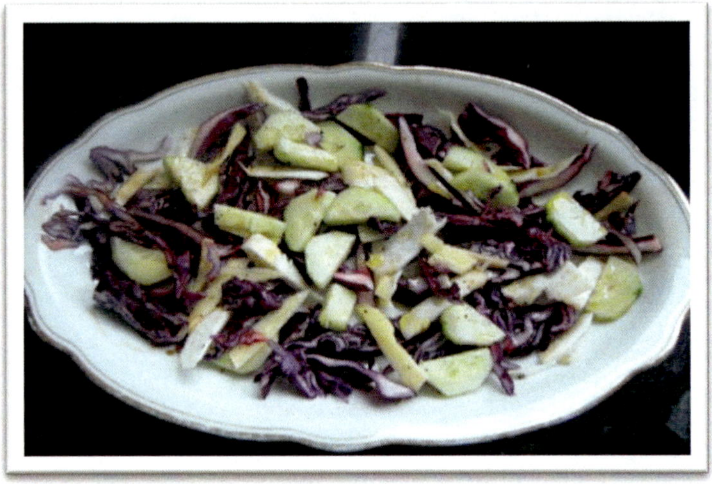

Side salad

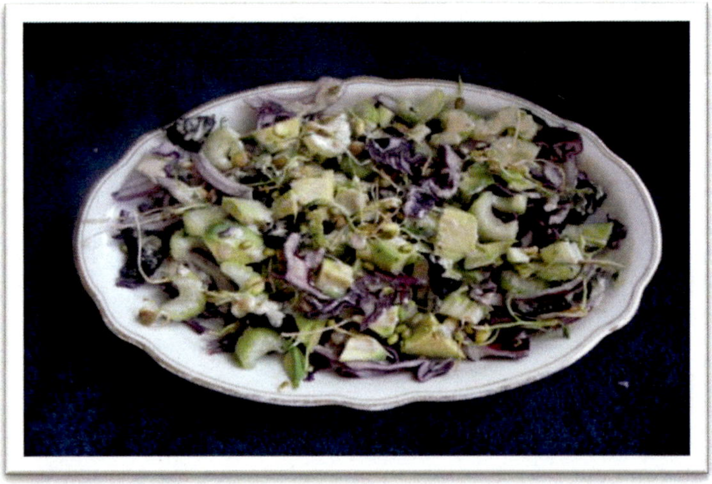

Pulse salad

Pulse salad

(see picture on page 94)

Ingredients:

½ cup sprouted mung beans

1 cup sprouted lentils

2 chopped spring onions

¼ red cabbage, thinly chopped

1 chopped avocado

3 tbsp raw almond butter

2 celery stalks chopped into small pieces

Dulse (sea vegetable)

Celtic sea salt (optional)

Black pepper (optional)

Preparation:

- Soak the mung beans and lentils in water overnight.
- Sieve and put into a bowl.
- Cut the avocado into small squares and add to the bowl. Add the onions, cabbage and celery.
- Now soak the dulse in water for 3-5 minutes then add it to the bowl.
- Mix the almond butter with water little by little until it forms a smooth sauce and pour on top of the salad. Enjoy!

EASY

Nutrition:

This salad is low in saturated fat and contains no cholesterol. It is high in dietary fibre, magnesium, iron, thiamin, potassium and very low in sodium. It also contains essential fatty acids vitamins A, C, beta-carotene, and protein.

SOUPS

Fresh carrot & avocado soup

(see picture on page 100)

Ingredients:

2 celery stalks

250 ml fresh carrot juice

1 large or 2 small avocado

1 clove garlic

Handful fresh coriander

1 tbsp extra-virgin olive oil

Sea salt, to taste (optional)

Black pepper

Preparation:

- Blend the celery stalks, carrot juice, avocado, and garlic clove on medium speed for 2 minutes until smooth.
- Add the olive oil and coriander and blend (leaving a little coriander for garnishing).
- Season with sea salt and black pepper to taste, if required.
- Before serving, garnish with some fresh coriander.

EASY

Nutrition:

Drinking this soup will support your immune system and promote good eyesight.

It is high in dietary fibre, vitamins A, C, K, potassium, folic acid, manganese, B6, calcium and magnesium and low in saturated fat and cholesterol.

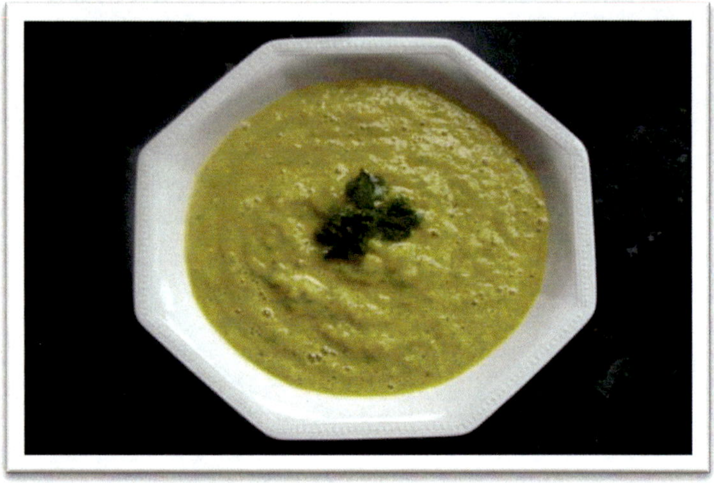

Fresh carrot & avocado soup

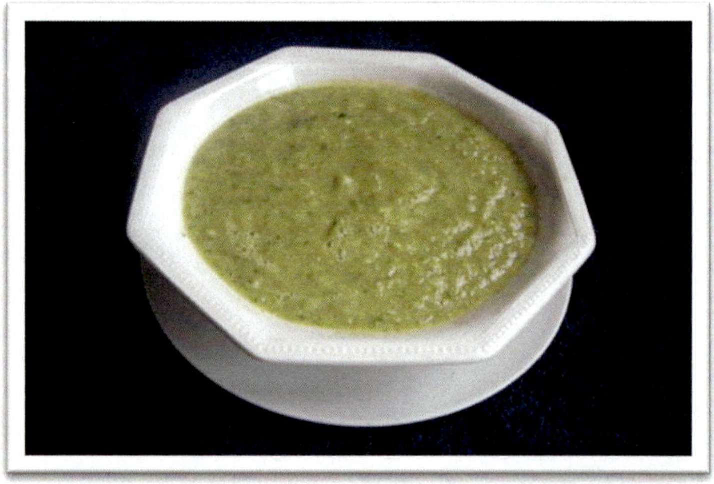

Easy sweet potato soup

Easy sweet potato soup

(see picture on page 100)

Ingredients:

2 medium sweet potatoes, chopped into small cubes

1 large leek, sliced into rings

2 tbsp of olive oil

1 avocado

Vegetable stock

Celtic salt and black pepper to taste, if required

Fresh watercress (to garnish)

Preparation:

- Cook the vegetables (apart from the avocado) with olive oil over medium heat for about 5 minutes.
- Add the vegetable stock and water enough to cover the contents and cook for 10-15 minutes until soft.
- Remove the contents and put in the blender together with the peeled avocado and blend to a creamy texture. You can now add the Celtic salt and black pepper, if required.
- Serve with shredded watercress to garnish.

EASY

Nutrition:

This dish is a good source of beta-carotene and antioxidants that lower risk of heart disease, diabetes and some types of cancer. It is a good source of dietary fibre.

Watercress contains high levels of calcium, vitamins C, B1, B6, K and E, iron, magnesium, manganese, zinc and potassium.

Research has shown that a plant compound called phenylethyl isothiocyanate (PEITC) found in watercress may have the capacity to switch off a signal in the body and starve a tumour of vital blood and oxygen.

Riki's chilled tomato soup

(see picture on page 105)

Ingredients:

6 large, fresh tomatoes

1 good sized avocado

1 cup water (or more, if required)

1 tsp ground cumin

1 clove garlic

1 cup fresh basil leaves

Celtic sea salt (if required)

Preparation:

- Chop the tomatoes and avocado and puree in a blender along with the water.
- Strain the mixture over a bowl and throw away anything left in the strainer.
- Pour the mix back into the blender, add the cumin, garlic leaves, basil leaves and Celtic sea salt (if required) and puree until smooth.

This dish can be served as a starter and is wonderfully cool in summer.

EASY

Nutrition:

This dish is a great source of lycopene, which is an antioxidant and has anti-cancer properties. Adding the smallest quantity of oil (e.g. avocado or olive oil) will help the absorption of these properties.

It is also a good source of dietary fibre, vitamins A, C, niacin, B6, potassium, folic acid, and essential fatty acids.

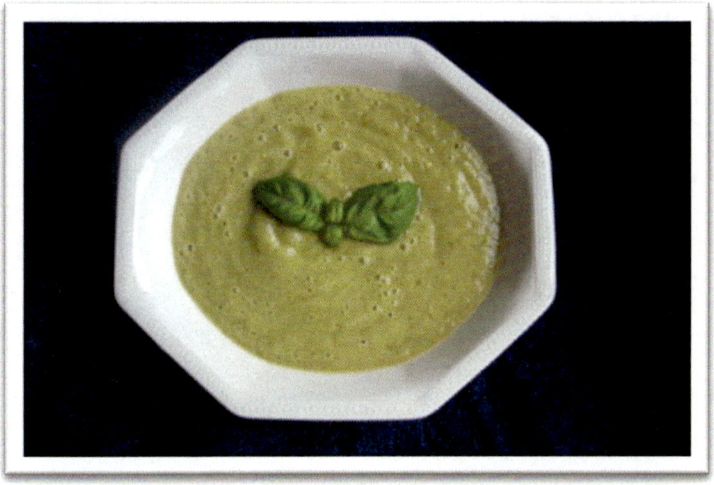

Riki's chilled tomato soup

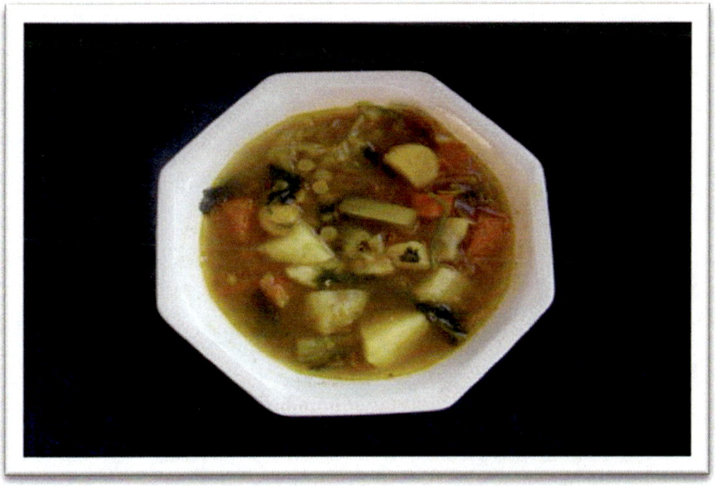

Riki's best vegetable soup

Fresh chilled avocado soup

Ingredients:

1 avocado

2 long celery sticks and some leaves

Handful watercress

Parsley

¼ tsp vegetable salt

Preparation:

- Blend all the above ingredients to a smooth consistency.
- Serve with some parsley on top to garnish.

This is a great soup for the summer season or just when you feel you need something uncooked and nutritionally preserved.

EASY

Nutrition:

This dish contains essential fatty acids, a high level of calcium, vitamin C, iron, B1, B6, K, E, magnesium, manganese, zinc and potassium. It is also a good source of dietary fibre.

Riki's best vegetable soup

(see picture on page 105)

Ingredients:

2 medium size potatoes
2 carrots
¼ pumpkin
1 onion
10 chestnuts
1-2 sweet potatoes
2 celery stalks and leaves
¼ green cabbage
1 courgette
30g red lentils
30g dhal
1-2 cubes vegetable stock
Black pepper
Turmeric
1 tablespoon olive oil
Fresh coriander
Water

Preparation:

- Peel the vegetables and cut into small cubes (cabbage can be cut into larger size).
- Put the olive oil in a large saucepan and swiftly fry the onion for one minute, add all the vegetables, lentils and dhal and leave the coriander aside.
- Mix together and add the water to cover the contents and leave to boil on a low heat.

- Add the stock, black pepper and turmeric and check after 20 minutes – if cooked to your satisfaction, add the coriander.
- Switch off the heat and leave the soup to simmer for 5-10 minutes.

This soup is quite filling, so you can freeze any left over for another time.

EASY

Nutrition:

An excellent source of dietary fibre, beta-carotene and proteins; low in calories, good source of folic acid, potassium and vitamins A and C; rich in minerals, vitamins and phyto-nutrients.

It is also a rich source of monounsaturated fatty acids that help reduce cholesterol.

Green lentil, leek & potato soup

(see picture on page 111)

Ingredients:

1 cup of green dry lentils

2 leeks

1 white potato

1 sweet potato

1 garlic clove (shredded)

2 tbsp olive oil

Vegetable stock

Celtic salt or vegetable salt & pepper to taste

Preparation:

- Soak the lentils for one hour prior to cooking.
- Wash and prepare all the vegetables, cutting the leeks into rings and the potatoes into cubes.
- In a large saucepan lightly fry the shredded garlic clove and add the lentils, leeks and potatoes and give it a quick stir to mix.
- Add enough water and vegetable stock to cover the contents and cook on a medium heat for 20 minutes and check if soft, otherwise give an extra 10 minutes.
- When almost ready, add the seasoning, and serve.

If you wish to make this dish thicker and creamier, put some of the ingredients in a blender until smooth, then stir the mix back in with the rest of the soup and enjoy!

EASY

Nutrition:

This dish is a good source of proteins.

Leek contains amounts of kaemfferol that protects blood vessel linings from damage and is known as a cardiovascular supporting vegetable.

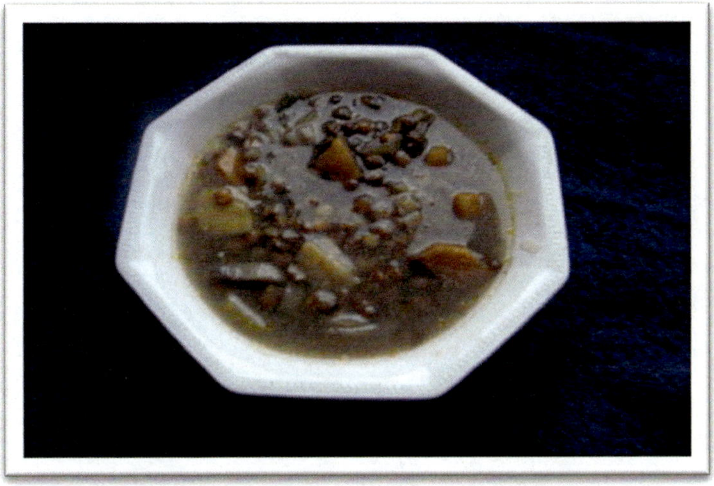

Green lentil, leek & potato soup

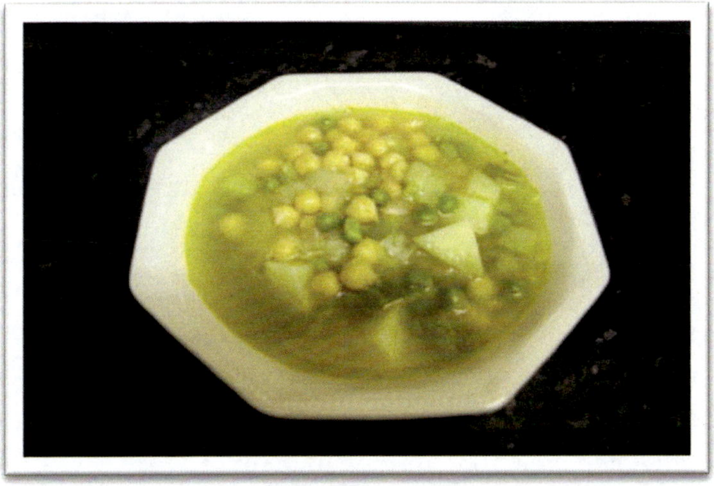

Winter soup

Winter soup

(see picture on page 111)

Ingredients:

1 potato

1 cup dried chickpeas

1 leek

2 tbsp olive oil

1 cup fresh or frozen peas

Vegetable stock

Celtic sea salt (optional)

Black pepper

¼ tsp red paprika

½ tsp Asafoetida yellow powder (optional)

Preparation:

- Soak the chickpeas overnight, drain and wash a couple of times.
- In a large saucepan add the olive oil and lightly fry the leek on a low heat.
- Cut the potato and add to the saucepan.
- Now add the chickpeas, peas and vegetable stock and fill with water to cover the contents and cook for ½ an hour.
- Add the Asafoetida, red paprika, black pepper and salt (if required) and cook for a further 10 minutes.
- Take off the heat and let the soup cool slightly for 10 minutes before serving.

EASY

Nutrition:

This soup is full of nutrients for the brain and body. It is low in fat and calories, and contains vitamins C, B1 and B6, folic acid, potassium, magnesium, calcium, fibre, carbohydrates, copper, zinc, iron, sodium, thiamin, riboflavin, niacin and essential fatty acids. Asafoetida yellow powder helps to expel flatulence.

Healthy soup for the soul

Ingredients:

¼ pumpkin

4 fresh tomatoes

1 cup dried chickpeas

1 medium size onion

¼ cup red or green lentils

Handful of fresh coriander

Celtic salt or vegetable seasoning to taste

Black pepper

2 tbsp olive oil

1 tsp ground turmeric

Preparation:

- Soak chickpeas in water overnight and drain before cooking.
- In a large saucepan quickly fry the onion in the olive oil then stir in the spices.
- Add the chickpeas, lentils and tomatoes and keep stirring for 5 minutes on a low heat.
- Add the rest of the chopped vegetables and mix together.
- Add enough water to cover the contents and leave to cook on a low to medium heat for 20-30 minutes – if the chickpeas are not soft enough, leave to cook for a further 10 minutes.
- Let the soup cool for a further 5 minutes before serving.

EASY

Nutrition:

This dish is packed with vitamins, minerals, fibre and antioxidants (e.g. carotenoids, vitamin A, C, K and E). It contains magnesium, potassium and iron, is a source of source of proteins and has anti-cancer properties.

Watercress soup

Ingredients:

1 tbsp olive oil

1 good size avocado

2-3 bunches watercress

4 Jerusalem artichokes

Vegetable or chicken stock

1 leek (sliced)

2 cloves garlic

250 ml water

Preparation:

- Heat the oil in a saucepan and gently fry the garlic and leek for about one minute.
- Add the vegetable/chicken stock and bring to the boil.
- Add the Jerusalem artichoke and watercress and simmer for about 3 minutes. Season with Celtic salt and freshly ground black pepper and allow to cool slightly.
- Put in a blender – you can now add the avocado and eat the soup warm, or let the mixture cool then add the avocado and eat it as cold, nutritious soup.

EASY

Nutrition:

Watercress contains high levels of calcium, vitamins C, B1, B6, K and E, iron, magnesium, manganese, zinc and potassium.

Research has shown that a plant compound called phenylethyl isothiocyanate (PEITC) found in watercress may have the capacity to switch off a signal in the body and starve a tumour of vital blood and oxygen.

Contains essential fatty acids

DRESSINGS, SAUCES, DIPS

Mum's best hummus

(see picture on page 122)

Ingredients:

1 cup dried chickpeas

3 tbsp tahini paste

¼ cup fresh lemon juice

4 tbsp extra virgin olive oil

4 cloves garlic, minced

Celtic sea salt to taste

Red paprika

Preparation:

- Soak the dried chickpeas in water overnight.
- Drain and cook until soft.
- Blend the chickpeas and all other ingredients in a blender apart from the tahini paste, salt and paprika.
- Mix the tahini with cold water until it becomes smooth and changes to a lighter colour.
- Add the tahini and salt to the rest of the combined ingredients and mix together.
- When serving, spread the hummus on a plate and drizzle with olive oil and a little of the red paprika.

This can be eaten with oatmeal crackers and green salad. You can also eat hummus as a dip with bite-size pieces of cucumber, celery, carrots and peppers (red and green).

EASY

Nutrition:

Chickpeas are rich in folic acid, manganese, tryptophan, copper, iron, and protein. Their high folic acid and tryptophan content make them particularly good for women of child-bearing age. They also aid restful sleep.

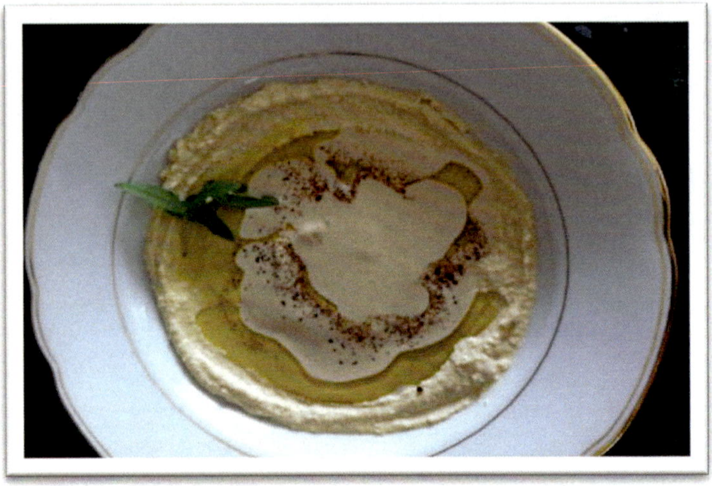

Mum's best hummus

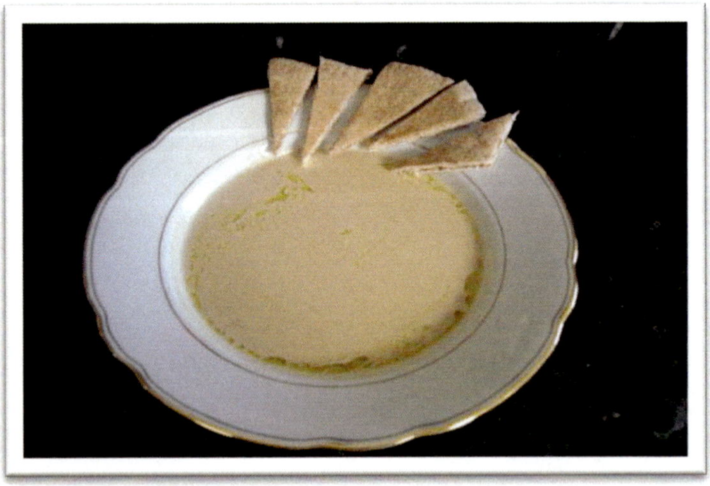

Riki's extra-zingy tahini paste

Riki's extra-zingy tahini paste

(see picture on page 122)

Ingredients:

3 tbsp tahini paste

Juice of ½ lemon

3 garlic cloves

Celtic or sea salt to taste

Water

1 tbsp olive oil

Preparation:

- Place the tahini paste, lemon juice and some of the water in a bowl and mix well; add more water as necessary until the paste changes to a lighter colour.
- Add the crushed garlic and salt to taste and mix together.
- Sprinkle with olive oil and serve.

This mix can be eaten with hummus, salad, falafel and wholemeal pitta bread or with oat crackers. Tahini can also be added to salad as a dressing or served as a dip with bite-size vegetables.

EASY

Nutrition:

Contains vitamins B1, B2, B3, B5 and B15 to promote healthy cell growth/division and prevent anaemia, and enhance immune and nervous system functions. B vitamins help protect the body against pancreatic cancer.

Tahini contains a high level of calcium. Just 35g will provide you with 1/3 of the recommended daily intake.

Nutty dip

(see picture on page 127)

Ingredients:

100g cashew nuts

100g macadamia nuts

100g sunflower seeds

3 tbsp fresh lemon juice

3 cloves of garlic

Handful fresh parsley

A little grated black pepper to taste

Pinch of Celtic sea salt (if required)

1 cup water

Preparation:

- Put all the ingredients in a food processor and little by little add the water until it forms a paste.
- Place the paste into a container and keep in the fridge (this paste can be kept for 3-4 days).

This dish can be served with chopped celery, carrots, cucumber, peppers (green and red) and would be great as a snack if you are on the move and very busy.

EASY

Nutrition:

This paste is rich in magnesium, copper, zinc, potassium, iron and selenium and is a good source of dietary fibre. It is of health promoting phytochemicals to protect against cancer and strokes.

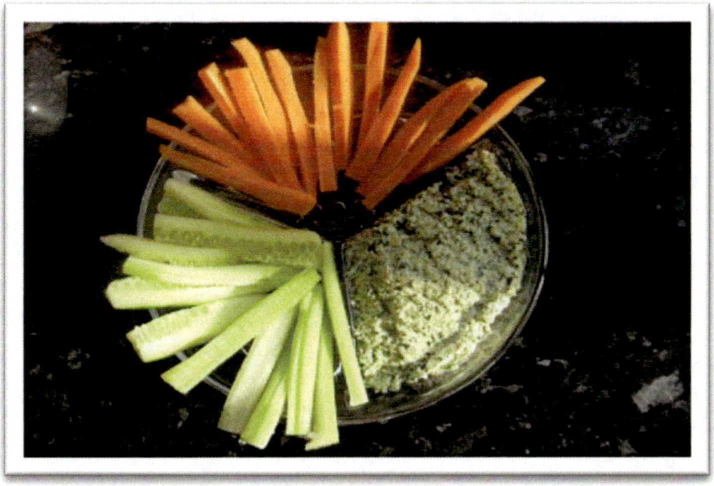

Nutty dip

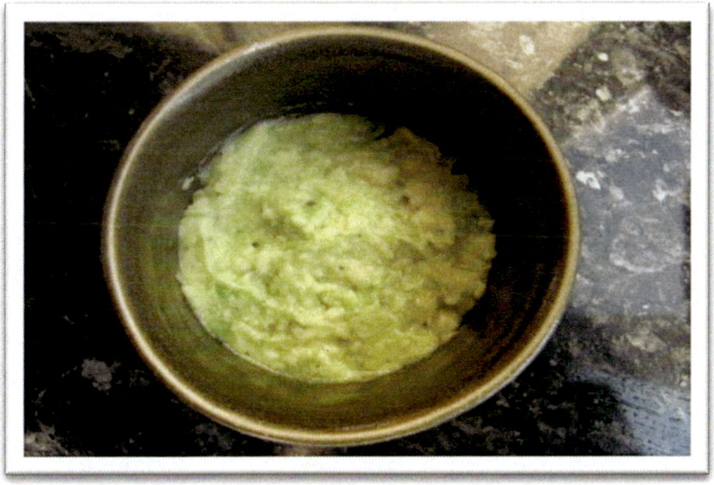

Riki's avocado dip

Riki's avocado dip

(see picture on page 127)

Ingredients:

2 avocados

Juice of 1 fresh lemon

Celtic sea salt

Black pepper

Olive oil (optional)

Preparation:

- Peel the avocados, place them in a dish and mash with a fork.
- Add the lemon juice, salt, black pepper and olive oil.

You can serve this as a dip with celery and carrot sticks or with crackers.

EASY

Nutrition:

This dish is full of essential fatty acids. It contains nearly twenty vitamins and minerals and phytonutrients including potassium, fibre, B-vitamins, folic acid and vitamin E.

DESSERTS

Mixed oatcake crackers & banana ice

(see picture on page 132)

Ingredients:

4 oatcake crackers

1 tsp Stevia granulated sugar or Manuka honey

3 tbsp elderberry juice

250g mixed berries

1 frozen banana

½ tsp cinnamon

Water

Preparation:

- Place the mixed fruit in a bowl; add the Stevia sugar or honey, elderberry juice, cinnamon and mix together. Leave to rest for 5 minutes.
- Place the oat crackers on a dessert plate and prepare the banana ice by putting the banana in an ice-cream maker or juicer, adding a small amount of water (to remove some of the ice freeze on the banana), and blending until it resembles ice-cream.
- Put the banana ice on the oat crackers, top with the mixed fruits and serve.

EASY

Nutrition:

Banana ice is a very refreshing alternative to ice cream without the need for dairy products. It is a good source of dietary fibre that helps lower blood cholesterol and control sugar levels.

Oats contain a phytoestrogen compound, which has been linked to a decreased risk of hormone related diseases like breast cancer. Oats are also a source of carbohydrates that provide calories for energy needs and contain a higher concentration of well-balanced protein not found in other types of breakfast cereal.

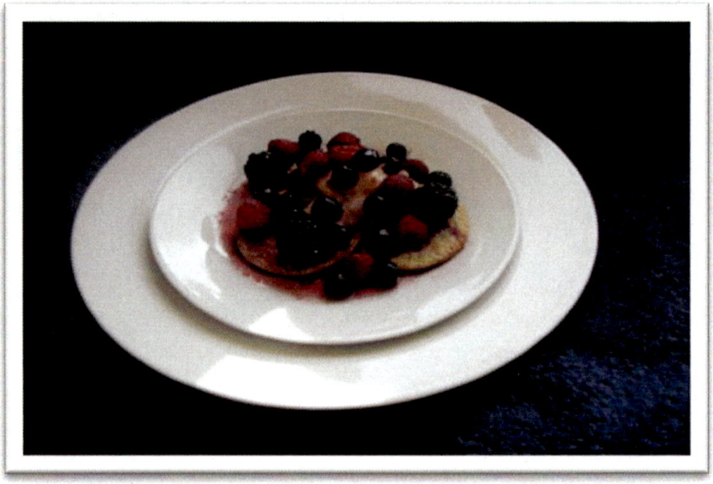

Mixed oatcake crackers & banana ice

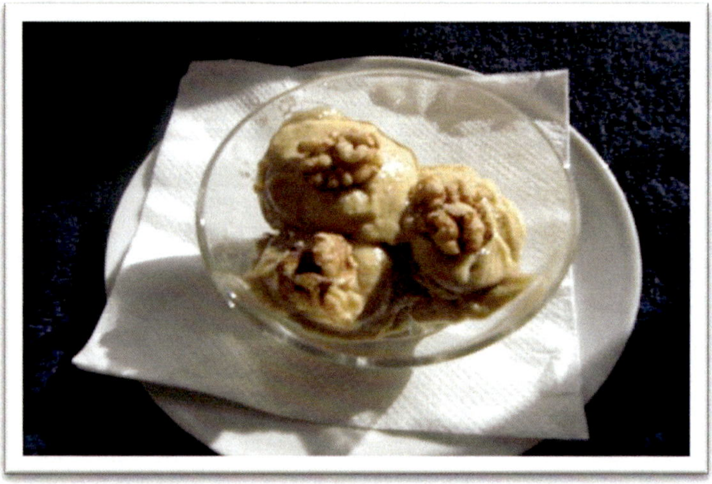

Mango, banana & walnut ice cream

Coco nibs biscuits

Ingredients:

2-3 tbsp organic coco nibs
1 star of anis, grated
2 cups buckwheat powder
3 tbsp raw almond or walnut butter
2 tbsp Stevia granulated sugar
1 tbsp coconut oil

Preparation:

- Place all ingredients, except the coco nibs, in a blender and blend to a smooth texture.
- Add the coco nibs and mix with wooden spoon.
- Preheat oven to a medium heat and put the coconut oil on the tray and spread.
- Shape the biscuits, place on the tray and bake in oven for 15-20 minutes.
- Cool and serve with ice cream made from natural frozen fruit or you can serve these biscuits without ice cream.

EASY

Nutrition:

These biscuits contain antioxidants, which protect against disease. They are a good source of potassium, calcium, magnesium, vitamins E, C, D, A, B1, and essential fatty acids, are low in saturated fat, and very low in cholesterol and sodium. They are also a good source of dietary fibre, copper and manganese.

Iced banana pie

Any good quality juicer can also be an ice cream maker (see **Useful Links** on page 317).

Ingredients:

3-5 bananas	½ cup dried coconut
1 pack dry almonds	3 dates (fresh, preferably)

Preparation:

- Using a little water, make a syrup from the dates and set aside.
- Put the peeled bananas in the freezer for 8 hours.
- Blend the almonds for approximately 30 seconds until they reach a powdery texture; remove and place in a bowl.
- Add dried coconut and mix together to be able to prepare a reasonable size crust.
- Gently add the syrup to the mix until thick enough to form a crust and spread evenly into a pie tray.
- Now remove the frozen bananas from the freezer.
- Position the juicer or icemaker towards the centre of the pie tray.
- Water the bananas slightly and place in the juicer; let the iced banana fall onto the crust and spread evenly over the mix.

This pie can be served immediately after preparation or alternatively place in the freezer, as long as you take it out at least ½ hour before serving.

EASY

Nutrition:

This dish is low in saturated fat and cholesterol. It is a good source of dietary fibre, vitamins C and A, potassium, manganese, vitamin B6, calcium, magnesium, proteins, zinc, folic acid, iron, essential fatty acids, antioxidants and flavonoids such as beta-carotene. It also contains phytonutrients such as vitamin E that help against cardiovascular disease and even cancer.

Mango, banana & walnut ice cream

(see picture on page 132)

Ingredients

2 mangoes

2 bananas

½ cup walnuts

Preparation:

- Cut the mangoes and bananas into 2.5 cm x 2.5 cm cubes; put in a container and place in the freezer for at least 8-24 hours prior to preparation.
- When ready put the bananas, mangoes and some of the walnuts into a blender.
- Add one tablespoon of water and blend for a minute, stop the blender and add the rest of the walnuts.
- Now make the ice cream into a ball shape, place in a dish and enjoy!

EASY

Nutrition:

This ice cream is a great source of dietary fibre, vitamins, minerals and antioxidants (vitamins A, beta-carotene, C, E and B6).

It is a good source of protein, low in saturated fat and cholesterol, and contains potassium, magnesium, calcium and zinc.

Marrow cake special bake

(see picture on page 141)

Ingredients:

2 full cups of grated marrow

(you can also make this cake with courgettes)

2 eggs

3 tbsp honey or Stevia granulated sugar

1 cup organic barley flour

1/3 tsp baking powder

½ tsp baking soda

¼ tsp Celtic salt

2 tsp grated cinnamon

1 tsp vanilla extract or 1 vanilla bean

1 cup chopped walnuts

½ cup coconut or vegetable oil

Water – if necessary

Dried coconut – optional

Preparation:

- Preheat oven to 220°C degrees. Use 1 tbsp of the coconut or vegetable oil to grease a baking tray (22.5 x 12.5 cm or bigger if needs be) and leave aside.
- Place all the ingredients in a bowl and mix rapidly (add a little water at this point, if necessary, and keep mixing).
- Spread the mixture evenly onto the baking tray and place in the pre-heated oven for 30-35 minutes.
- Remove from the oven, sprinkle some dried coconut on top, and leave to cool before serving.

EASY

Nutrition:

This is a good source of dietary fibre, vitamins C and A, essential fatty acids, magnesium, zinc and proteins, and a rich supply of flavonoids that protect against disease.

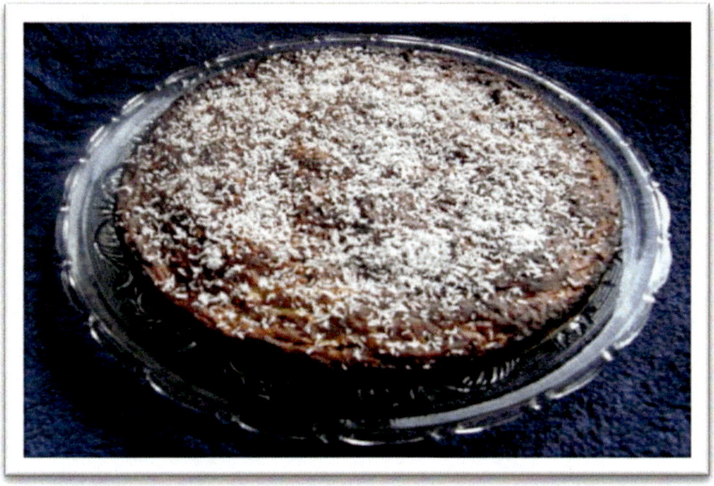

Marrow cake special bake

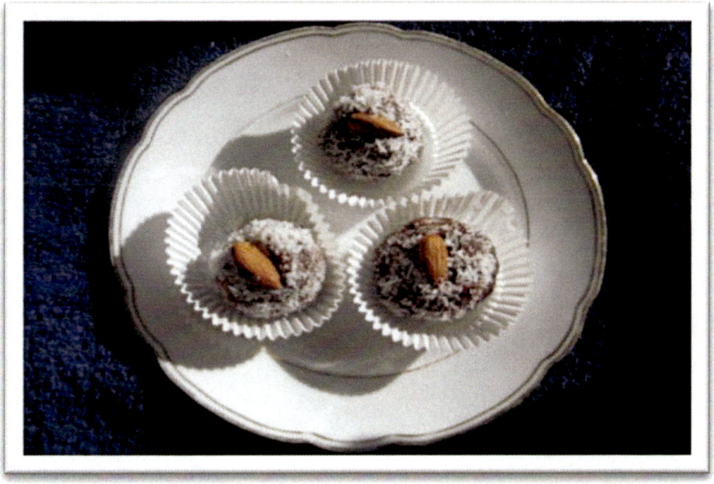

Real natural choc balls

Real natural choc balls

(see picture on page 141)

Ingredients:

2 tsp organic raw cocoa powder

10-12 dates

¼ cup pine nuts

2 tbsp dried coconut

¼ cup almonds

½ cup walnuts

Warm water

Preparation:

- Combine dates and warm water and leave aside to soften.
- Place the pine nuts and walnuts in a blender on a medium speed until almost powdery but not a paste.
- Add the cocoa powder and start adding the dates little by little until you get nice texture and enough to be able to hold it in your hand and roll to a ball.
- Now spread the dried coconut on a plate and start making 5 cm x 5 cm balls and then roll them in the plate to cover in the dried coconut, place them on a separate plate and put one almond on top of each choc ball.

These can be stored in the fridge for almost a week.

These are nutritious, full of vitamins and minerals and completely natural.

EASY

Nutrition:

This is low in cholesterol and sodium, and a good source of protein, potassium, zinc, iron, magnesium, essential fatty acids, calcium and vitamin E.

Dishy carob dessert

Ingredients:

1 cup almonds

1 cup walnuts

1 cup pine nuts

1 avocado

¾ cup carob powder

½ cup organic cocoa powder

Stevia granulated sugar to taste (optional)

Preparation:

- Soak the almonds and walnuts for 5 hours; sieve and put in a blender.
- Add the pine nuts and mix for 30 seconds.
- Add the carob powder, cocoa powder, avocado and some of the Stevia (optional) and mix for a further 20 seconds.
- Add 2-3 tablespoons of water to form the mix.
- Make 5 cm x 5 cm cubes and place in a small dish and decorate each one with a small piece of walnut.
- Place in the fridge to set (any excess can be stored in the freezer for another time).

EASY

Nutrition:

This dessert is a good source of protein, vitamins A, B, B2, B3, and D, and has a high level of calcium, phosphorus, potassium, magnesium and iron. It is also an excellent source of fibre, vitamin E and folic acid.

Orange & cinnamon dessert

(see picture on page 148)

Ingredients:

Juice of 1 freshly squeezed orange

Juice of ½ lime

2 avocados

½ tsp cinnamon

Stevia granulated sugar to taste

Pinch of Celtic salt (optional)

A little grated lime (for decoration)

Mint leaves (for decoration)

Preparation:

- Prepare the orange juice and set aside.
- Peel or scoop the avocados and put in a blender.
- Add all other ingredients, including the orange and lime juices, and mix quickly to form a delicious smooth texture.
- Divide into dessert cups, sprinkle with grated lime and decorate with mint leaves.
- Keep in the fridge until time to serve.

EASY

Nutrition:

This dessert is a great source of dietary fibre, vitamin C, calcium, iron, vitamin K and manganese. It aids digestion and boosts energy.

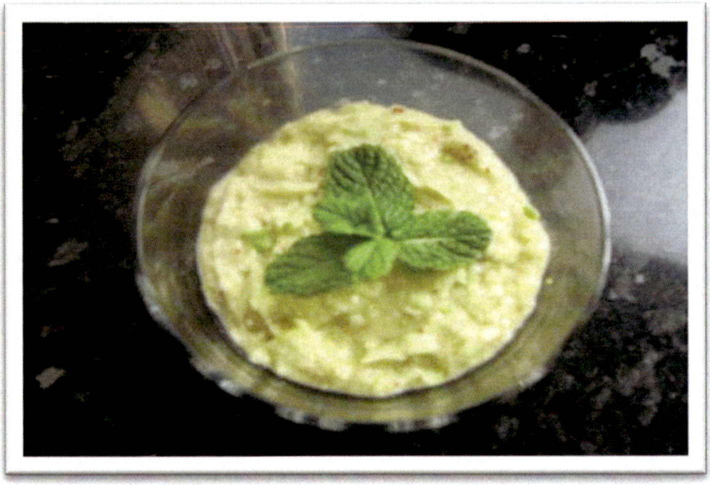

Orange & cinnamon dessert

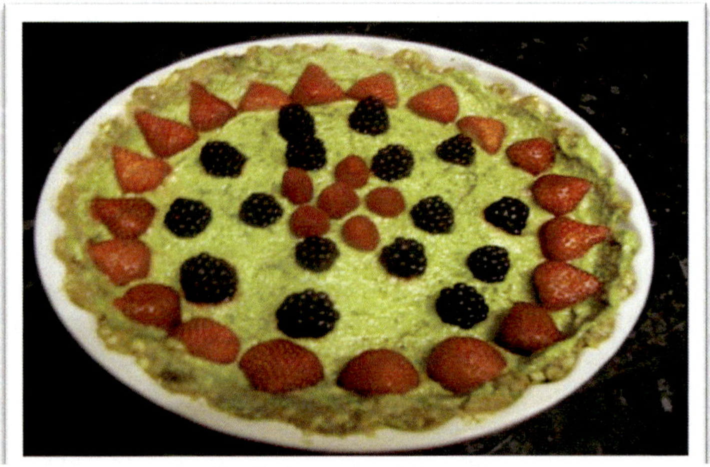

Delicious healthy pie

Delicious healthy pie

(see picture on page 148)

Ingredients:

1 good sized avocado	10 fresh dates
1 cup almonds	2 cups shredded dried coconut
1 cup cashew nuts	1-2 tbsp orange or lime juice
1 cup sunflower seeds	Grated lime
Pinch of Celtic salt (optional)	2-3 tbsp Manuka honey

Preparation:

- Place the almonds, cashew nuts, sunflower seeds, ½ of the dried coconut and a pinch of salt in a blender and mix for 30 seconds.
- Add the fresh dates and mix for a further 10 seconds.
- Remove and place in a pie dish and squeeze the contents into the bottom and side of the dish until evenly spread.

Prepare the filling:

- Place the peeled avocado, the orange or lime juice, the remaining dry coconut and the Manuka honey in the blender and mix together briefly.

- Fill the pie with the contents and spread the grated lime on top. Decorate with fruits and place in the fridge (or the freezer if you wish to keep it for longer).
- This dish is best eaten when chilled for at least 5-6 hours.

EASY

Nutrition:

This dish is a great source of dietary fibre, proteins, essential fatty acids, zinc, folic acid and antioxidant. It can help lower cholesterol. It is also a source of carbohydrates (containing 80% natural sugar), vitamin B6, thiamin, niacin, and certain amino acids, calcium, copper, iron, magnesium, manganese, phosphorus, potassium, and sodium, and has antibacterial properties.

Apple & courgette pie

(see picture on page 153)

Ingredients:

2 medium size courgettes

1 cup mixed nuts (almonds, pine nuts, cashew nuts)

1 tsp Stevia granulated sugar

1 cooking apple

½ cup goji berries

½ cup dried coconut

10 fresh dates

2 tbsp lime juice

Grated lime peel

¼ tsp mixed spice of clove & cinnamon

Preparation:

- Form the pie crust by blending the mixed nuts, dried coconut and fresh dates.
- Remove the mixture and press down evenly onto the base and the sides of the pie dish.
- Put in the freezer to set for 10-15 minutes.
- Grate the courgette and apple, add the lime juice and mix together; add the mixed spice, Stevia and goji berries and fill the pie.
- Sprinkle the grated lime peel on top of the pie.
- Keep in the freezer for one hour prior to serving and leave in the freezer if you wish to keep it longer.

EASY

Nutrition:

This dish is a great source of dietary fibre and contains no saturated fat or cholesterol. It contains vitamin C and beta-carotene (as powerful antioxidants), B-complex, B6, some potassium, phosphorus and calcium and is a source of folic acid.

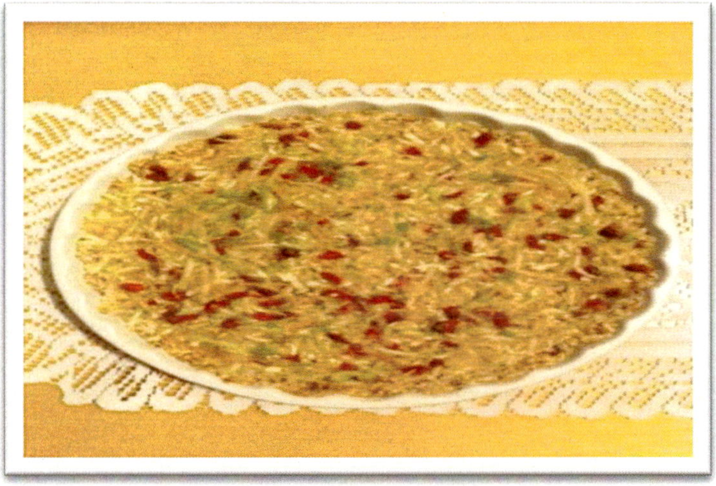

Apple & courgette pie

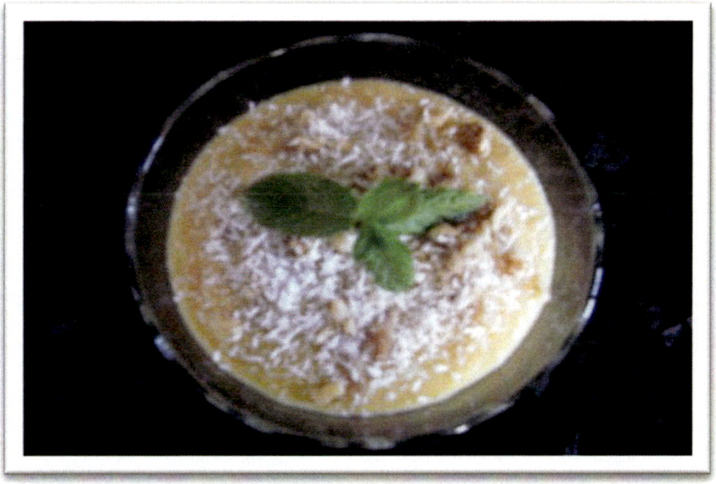

Banana & mango mousse

Banana & mango mousse

(see picture on page 153)

Ingredients:

1 banana

1 mango

1 tsp Stevia granulated sugar

2 tbsp lucuma powder

½ tsp vanilla essence or fresh pod

2 tbsp coconut butter

2 tbsp rose water

10g grated walnuts

10g dried coconut

Mint leaf (for decoration)

Preparation:

- Prepare the banana and mango and put in a blender; add Stevia sugar and blend to a smooth texture.
- Add the vanilla, coconut butter, rose water and the lucuma powder and mix for a further 30 seconds.
- Serve in small dishes, sprinkle with grated walnuts and dried coconut. Decorate with the mint leaf.
- Put in the fridge until serving.

EASY

Nutrition:

This dish is a source of dietary fibre, protein, zinc, vitamin A, beta-carotene, vitamins C, E and B6, potassium, magnesium, and calcium.

HOW TO GROW YOUR OWN PRODUCE

Aduki beans – V*igna angularis*

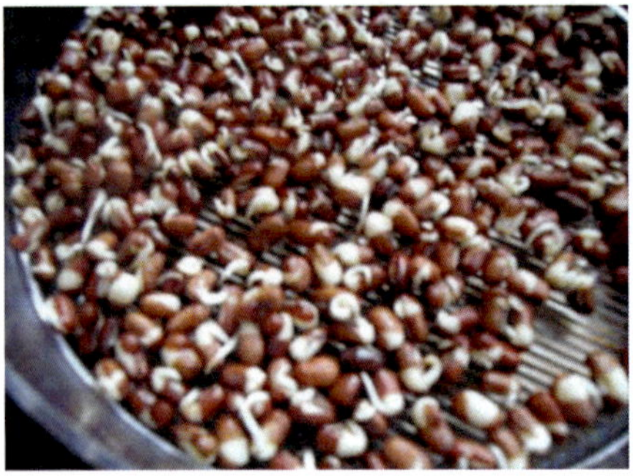

Aduki beans are small, reddish-brown beans with a white ridge along one edge. They have a sweet, nutty flavour when cooked. The two kinds of aduki beans are (1) Hokkaido, which are round, shiny, and a deep maroon colour and are grown in Japan, and (2) Aduki, which are smaller and lighter in colour and less sweet. These are grown in the United States as well as in Asia.

Properties and medicinal uses: Aduki beans help keep bowel movements regular and fortify the kidneys. They are a good source of energy, and also help lower cholesterol. In some quarters it is believed they may play a role in preventing breast cancer. Aduki beans are high in protein and low in fat. They also contain high levels of potassium and fibre, the B vitamins, thiamin, niacin and riboflavin, and minerals such as iron, zinc, and manganese.

Planting time and harvesting: ***Sprouted aduki beans.*** Place the aduki beans in a clean jam jar; put a piece of netting or muslin over the top of the jar and secure in place (this will act as a sieve); water overnight or for at least 8 hours. Next day, sieve the water by inverting the jar, rinse the sprouts and replace with fresh water. In warm weather, rinse your sprouts twice daily, as they will become more easily dehydrated; in colder weather, once is usually enough. Be sure to drain well after each rinse. (It doesn't matter whether the jar is kept in light or shade at this stage, but direct sunlight is best avoided.)

Repeat this process every day for 4-5 days until the shoots begin sprouting. This is when you can start using them in salads on a daily basis. When your sprouts are ready they should be kept in an airtight container (their original jar will suffice) and kept in the fridge. This way further growth is inhibited and they will stay fresh for 3-4 days.

Part used: Beans

Preparation: May be eaten cooked or raw in salads, before or after they produce the shoots, or juiced for their nutritious benefit.

Recommended consumption: For maximum benefit from aduki beans, half a cup per week should be consumed, and for those who are ill, half a cup twice a week.

Artichoke (globe) –*Cynara cardunculus*

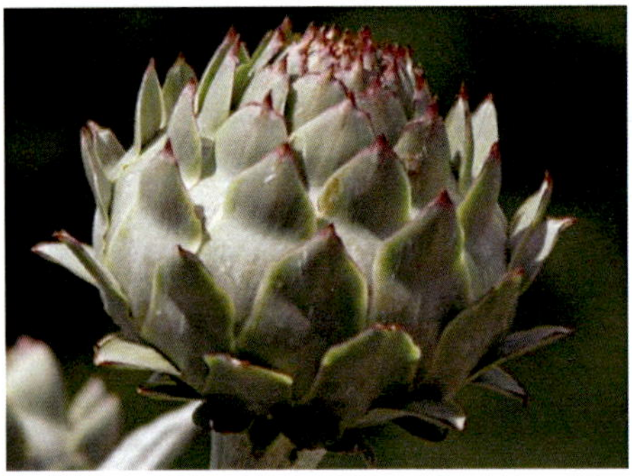

Copyright © 2005 Brunswyk

The artichoke is a perennial thistle, native to Southern Europe and the Mediterranean region.

Properties and medicinal uses: The artichoke is a bitter plant and is highly beneficial in treating liver disorders (detoxifies and regenerates liver tissues), and is useful if consumed prior to drinking alcohol, as a protection against hangovers. It stimulates the gall bladder and reduces blood sugar and cholesterol.

Planting time and harvesting: Planting should be carried out in April on a well-manured site. Allow a minimum of 70 cm around each plant. In May, mulch well and remove all flower heads in the first season. In autumn, remove all dead and dying leaves and protect the plants against frost. The following spring, feed with a general fertilizer at the rate of 2-3oz per square yard.

Begin cropping the flower heads in July (and before they start turning brown at the edges). The king Crown (the large central head) should be harvested first.

Globe artichokes crop best in the second and third years, so it is worthwhile replacing them every three years. Ideally, to achieve annual crops it is advisable to have three beds of varying ages in operation at any one time

Part used: Leaves, roots, flower head.

Preparation: Prepare the artichoke immediately before cooking by removing the top 2.5 cm of the head with a sharp knife. Trim back the stalk to within 2.5 cm of the bottom and remove any loose leaves. Clip off the tips of all other leaves. The heads are now ready for cooking.

Alternatively cut the leaves and clear the heart from the fibres, then cut into four pieces on the plate and sprinkle lemon, a pinch of sea salt, black pepper and a dash of olive oil. This is good to eat if you need a liver tonic. You can also put the whole globe into slightly salted boiling water for 20 minutes until the leaves change colour and can lift off the plant easily. Do not spoil the leaves as you can eat the top, tender part of it, then remove the centre and eat the heart of the plant. Artichoke can be served hot or cold as salad.

Asparagus – *Asparagus officinalis*

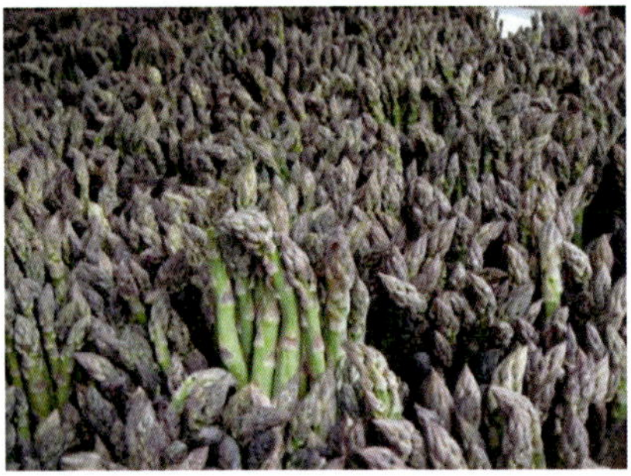

Asparagus, a perennial plant that appears in springtime, has spear-like, edible shoots. It develops on rhizomes (a mass of horizontal roots). This vegetable is native to Europe and eastern Asia.

Properties and medicinal uses: Asparagus is a bitter, cleansing herb that is particularly beneficial for the bowels, liver and kidneys. It can be taken internally for cystitis, gout, kidney disease, oedema (from heart failure) and rheumatism.

Planting time and harvesting: As asparagus is a long-term crop, good preparation of the plot is crucial. Whilst it can be grown from seed, it is more common to plant 1-2 year old seedling crowns. These are usually planted in 120 cm wide beds with 3 rows to a bed, the crowns being 45 cm apart in each row.

Dig a trench 20-25 cm deep and 30 cm wide. Make a small ridge along the bottom of this trench and place the crowns on this ridge with the string like roots spread out evenly on each side of the ridge. Then cover with about 7.5-10 cm of soil.

As you hoe during the growing season, gradually fill in the trench. And twice-yearly, in autumn and spring, draw up the earth over the rows in the same manner as you would for potatoes.

In spring, use an organic fertilizer to feed the bed and mulch well in the autumn with well-rotted manure or compost (preferably organic). Top growth should be cut off in November.

Do not harvest the asparagus spears until the second year of growth. You can then harvest all available shoots over a four-week period – this will extend to six weeks in subsequent years.

Harvest by cutting the spears 5-7.5 cm below the surface of the bed when the shoots are approximately 12.5 cm high, thus giving a total spear length of approximately 17.5-20 cm. Trim off the tough ends and remove any large scales along the stalk. Wash carefully to remove all grit then tie into bunches.

Part used: Young shoots, rhizomes

Preparation: Spears should be steamed and served hot or cold as a vegetable, used in salad or in soup.

Beetroot – *Beta vulgaris*

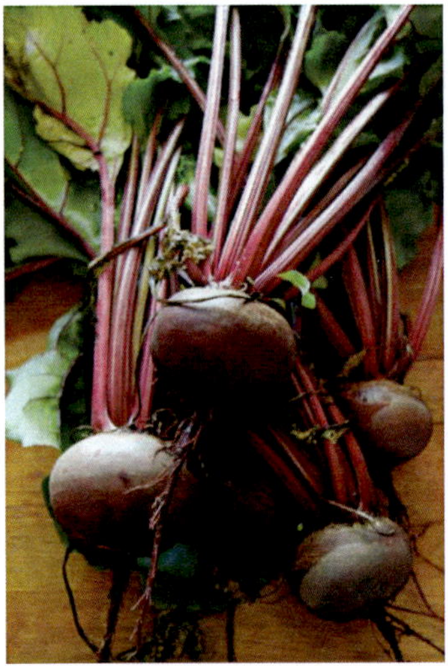

Beetroot comes in two types: (1) the round or globe beetroot, or (2) the long-rooted or tapering beet. The globe beetroot is probably best for early crops and the long-rooted beet for late crops and winter storage.

Properties and medicinal uses: Beetroot is very nutritious and a good source of magnesium, iron, phosphorus and vitamin B6. Betacyanin, the pigment that gives beetroot its colour, has significant antioxidant properties. Tests have shown beet fibre to have cholesterol lowering capabilities and the juice to lower blood pressure.

The bioactive agent betaine in beetroot supports healthy liver function and is thought to be a useful means to help prevent cancer. However, beetroot and beet greens contain high levels of oxalate, and should not be eaten by individuals with kidney stones containing oxalate.

Planting time and harvesting: Both types of beet have seeds that are small and knobbly and are actually small clusters of seeds. Prepare the ground by digging well and make drills 30 cm apart and 2.5 cm deep. The seed clusters should be planted 2 or 3 together with 15 cm between each planting. Beet can be sown from April-July to maintain a succession of roots. Lift the roots as required for immediate use.

In October lift all remaining roots and remove tops before storing in layers of sand in a shed or sheltered place. Remove all but about 4 cm of the tops. It is preferable to twist them off rather than cutting them with a knife and wash the root well. Uncover and use as required during the winter.

Part used: Root and young leaves.

Preparation: When cooked, drain the beetroot, plunge into cold water and rub off the skin. Small beetroots can be served whole and larger ones sliced or diced. Serve either hot or cold.

Marinate in lemon juice, black pepper, a pinch of Celtic salt, some cumin seeds or powder and olive oil.

Broad (fava) bean – *Vicia faba*

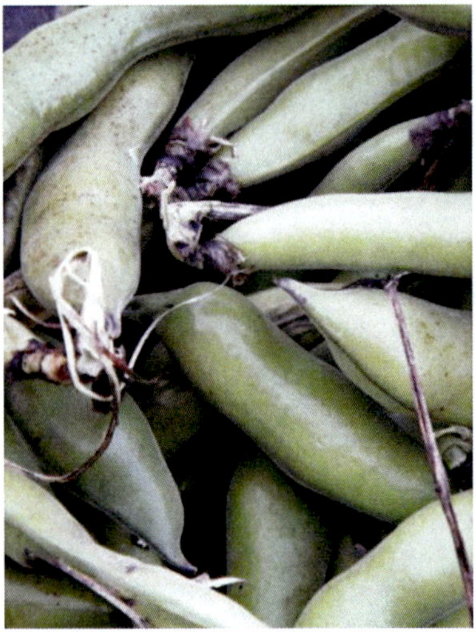

The leaves of the broad (or fava) bean are a grey-green colour and, unlike other vetches, do not have tendrils for climbing over other vegetation. The flowers have five black and white petals.

Properties and medicinal uses: Broad beans are rich in a substance called L-dopa, which is used in the clinical treatment of Parkinson's disease. L-dopa is also a natriuretic agent (the discharge of sodium through urine is known as *natriuresis*), which might help in controlling hypertension.

Planting time and harvesting: Broad beans are best consumed while still young and tender, so it is acceptable to begin harvesting as early as the middle of spring for plants started under glass or over-wintered in a sheltered location. If sown in early spring they will be ready from mid to late summer. The pods should be well filled, crisp, and a darkish-green colour, while the shelled bean should be plump with a tender skin, which is green to greenish white.

Prepare flat drills 7.5 cm deep and 15 cm wide, with rows 90 cm apart. Place the seeds 15 cm apart and staggered along the drill and cover.

Remove the growing tip of each plant when the plants have grown and there are a reasonable amount of young pods.

Part used: Beans.

Preparation: Broad beans take about 20 minutes to cook and can be used as a basic vegetable or an ingredient in a variety of other dishes. The young leaves of the plant can also be eaten either raw or cooked like spinach.

Broccoli – *Brassica oleracea*

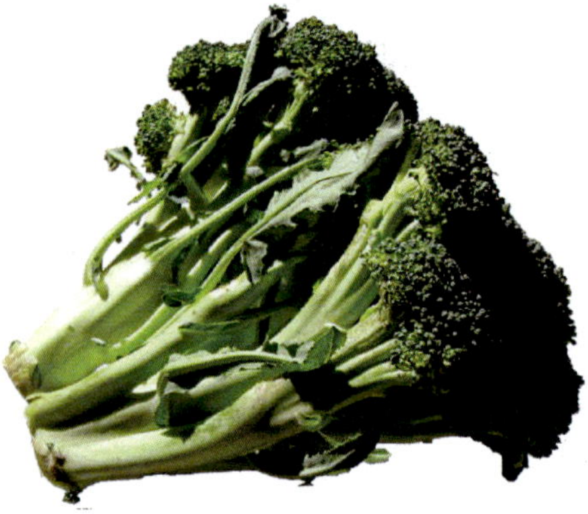

Copyright © 2005 David Monniaux

Broccoli is a member of the *Brassica* family (which includes cabbage, brussels sprouts, turnips, mustard and wallflowers) and is native to coastal southern and western Europe. It flourishes in rich, well-firmed soil and it is essential to prepare the site for the crops well in advance of planting.

Properties and medicinal uses: Broccoli is high in vitamin C, dietary fibre and contains many nutrients with powerful anti-cancer properties, e.g. diindolylmethane and a little selenium. It is also an excellent source of indole-3-carbinol, a chemical that enhances DNA repair in cells and appears to impede the growth of cancer cells. Broccoli has the highest levels of carotenoids in the brassica family. It is particularly rich in lutein (an antioxidant) and also provides beta-carotene (a primary dietary source of pro-vitamin A).

A high intake of broccoli has been found to reduce the risk of aggressive prostate cancer and its consumption has also been shown to be beneficial in the prevention of heart disease.

Planting time and harvesting: Broccoli seeds are very small and should be sown in shallow drills 13 mm deep with 15-23 cm between the rows. Sprinkle them thinly along the drill. Fill in the drills by shuffling the soil into them with the feet and treading down using even pressure, avoiding digging in the heels. The best months for sowing are March, April and May in order to give a reasonable succession of crops.

When the seedlings are about 10-15 cm high they are ready to be planted in specially prepared beds. Plant them very firmly every 60 cm along the rows, which should be 75 cm apart. When well established, give a top dressing of a good general organic fertilizer.

Harvest the broccoli before the flowers start to open (no yellow should be showing in the buds). Select broccoli that is fresh and clean with a firm but tender stalk. 1½ lbs will provide 4 good servings.

Part used: Flower heads and stem.

Preparation: Broccoli is often boiled but this reduces its health benefits. Try lightly steaming the vegetable or eating it raw.

Cabbage (green) – *Brassica oleracea*

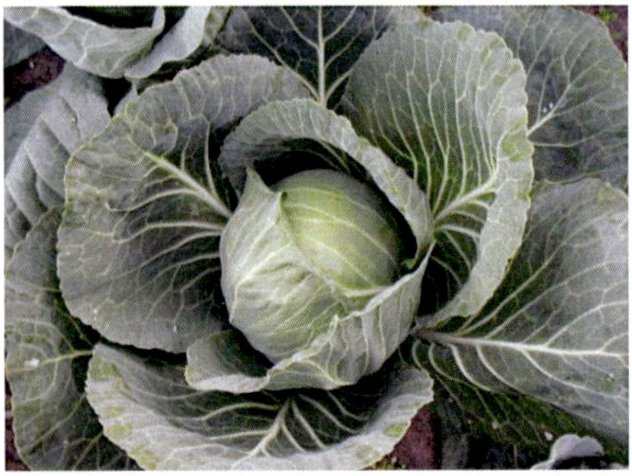

Green cabbage is one of the most popular types of cabbage. Choose green cabbage that has crisp, bright looking leaves without any holes or discoloured patches. It should be firm and heavy for its size.

Properties and medicinal uses: Cabbage is rich in phytonutrients, which work to protect the body from free radicals. Phytonutrients also signal our genes to increase production of enzymes (proteins that increase the rate of chemical reactions) involved in the detoxification process.

Cabbage may also lower the incidence of cancer, especially that of the lung, stomach, colon and prostate. Cabbage is a muscle builder, blood cleanser and eye strengthener. As a juice, fresh raw cabbage has been proved to heal stomach ulcers as well as being effective in treating fungus infection (due to its sulphur content). It can also lower serum cholesterol.

Planting time and harvesting: Sow the seeds on seed beds in drills 2 cm deep from April until July. When they are big enough, transfer the plants to the prepared beds with 45 cm between plants and rows. Ideally, cabbages should have reasonably solid heads and be heavy for their size.

Part used: The whole of the cabbage, minus the hard core.

Preparation: Remove any damaged outer leaves and cut the cabbage into small pieces, leaving the hard core to be disposed of. Wash thoroughly.

Cabbage can be steamed, boiled or stir-fried. However, it is easy to overcook cabbage and lose its nutritional value, so cook until it's just tender but still crisp. To steam cabbage, place in a steamer and cook for 5-10 minutes; to boil, bring a pan of water to the boil, add the prepared cabbage and cook for 5-8 minutes; to stir-fry, heat 1 tbsp olive oil in a frying pan, add the cabbage and stir-fry for 4-5 minutes.

Cabbage (red) – *Brassica oleracea var. capitata rubra*

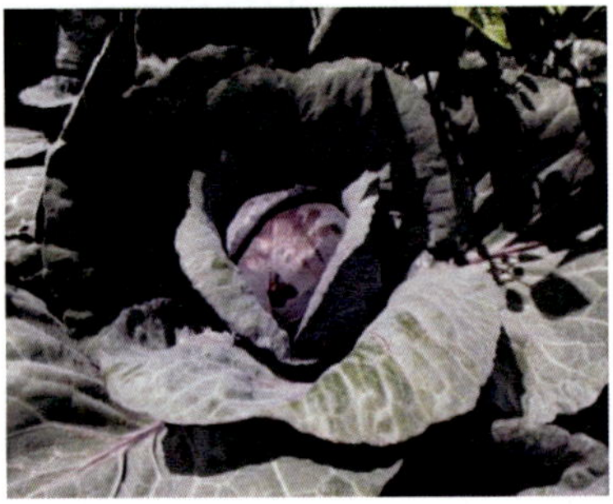

The leaves of the red cabbage are a purplish-dark red. However, an alkaline soil will produce greenish-yellow coloured cabbages. This explains the fact that the same plant is known by different colours in various regions.

Red cabbage requires well-fertilized soil and sufficient humidity to grow well, and is seeded in spring and harvested in late autumn.

Properties and medicinal uses: The red cabbage has more phytonutrients than the green cabbage, while the vitamin C content of red cabbage is 6-8 times higher than that of the green variety. Red cabbage also contains anthocyanin, which is an antioxidant that can help protect brain cells, and is believed to be an aid in the prevention of Alzheimer's disease.

Planting time and harvesting: Grow the red cabbage in exactly the same way as green cabbage. Ideally, start red cabbage seeds indoors 4 weeks before the last frost. Sow the seeds in spring and once the seedlings are about 5 cm tall and have their first leaves, they are ready to be moved outside for transplanting. Red cabbage prefers a moist and cool climate and can be placed in the ground while spring is still cool. The plants should be spaced about 30-60 cm apart. Although needing frequent watering, they are otherwise low-maintenance plants.

Part used: The whole of the cabbage, minus the hard core.

Preparation: On cooking, red cabbage will normally turn blue. However, to retain the red colour, just add vinegar or acidic fruit to the pot. Red cabbage is often used for salads and coleslaw. This vegetable can be eaten raw or cooked (like the green variety).

Carrots – *Daucus carota sativus*

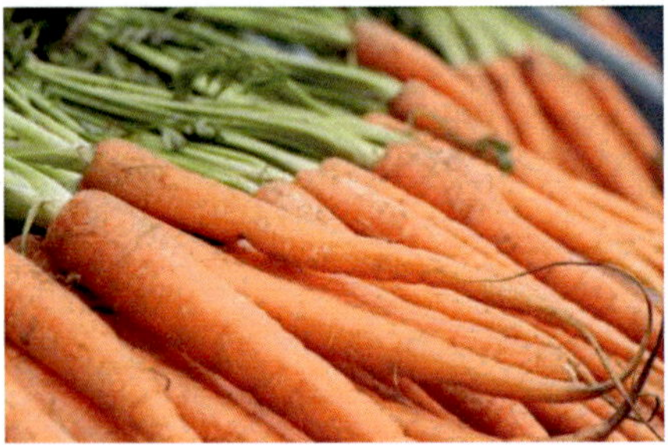

Carrots are a firm favourite with growers. The root of the carrot is packed with vitamin A or carotene and just 50g of raw carrot provides the body with the average daily requirement.

Carrots are a root crop and require a well-prepared but not recently manured ground. Most gardens are capable of producing a reasonable crop of carrots provided they are not too heavily shaded.

Properties and medicinal uses: Carrot contains vitamin A, which is essential for tissue growth, especially within the bones. Vitamin A is also very important for good vision as vitamin A deficiency can lead to problems such as night blindness. It is also essential for expectant mothers and the unborn foetus. However, it is also important to consume *moderate* levels of vitamin A, as too much can lead to liver toxicity and other health problems.

Carrot juice is a great source of vitamin C. A 227.5 ml glass of pure carrot juice can provide you with up to 35% of your daily recommended dosage of vitamin C. Pure carrot juice is also a very low calorie drink; a 227.5 ml glass being approximately 80 calories.

Planting time and harvesting: Sow the seeds thinly in drills 2 cm deep with 22 cm between the rows for stump-rooted varieties and 30 cm for other types of carrot.

The first sowings can be made in March/April with successive sowings being made until July. Seedlings should be thinned to 13 mm apart once big enough to handle. When the roots reach finger size, pull every other one for immediate use and allow the rest to grow on. A good crop of carrots should be brightly coloured and have firm flesh.

Part used: Being a rich source of vitamins, minerals and protein, the carrot root and the green leaves are both edible and highly nutritious. Carrot greens are also high in vitamin K, which is lacking in the carrot root.

Preparation: Carrots can be prepared whole, sliced, diced or shredded. Boil for 10-15 minutes and use as a side dish or a salad dish. They can also be added to soup or eaten raw or juiced. Carrots are also ideal for juicing. Try combining carrot and spinach to create a very rich source of vitamin A, or carrot and turnip for potassium (a 227.5 ml glass will provide up to 10% of your daily recommended level of potassium). However, if you suffer from a kidney disorder then you should avoid taking large amounts of potassium. Carrot and broccoli combined will provide you with a delicious vegetable calcium drink. A 227.5 ml glass will provide you with 6% of the daily recommended intake.

Celery – *Apium graveolens*

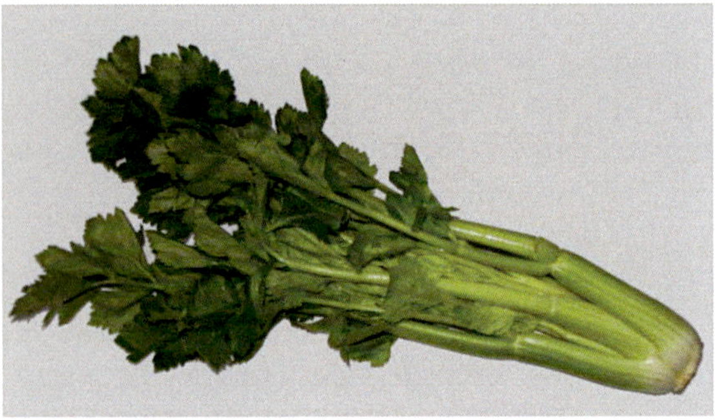

Copyright © 2005 Popolon

Celery is a wild plant that will grow practically anywhere. *Apium graveolens* is eaten as a vegetable either for the crisp leaf stalk or the fleshy top root.

Properties and medicinal uses: Celery acts as a blood purifier and is sometimes taken for arthritis. The low-calorie dietary fibre in celery is also useful in weight-loss diets, whilst celery seeds are a rich source of calcium and a good alternative to animal products.

Planting time and harvesting: Sow celery seeds in boxes in a heated greenhouse in March, with a further sowing in April to extend the growing season. When the seedlings are big enough to handle, prick out into boxes for growing on. In May-June, transplant then into a well-prepared cropping bed that has been dug deeply, incorporating plenty of manure or organic compost. Dig a trench 30-37.5 cm wide and deep, using more organic material in the base soil. Refill two thirds of the trench, leaving built up ridges on each side.

Place the celery plants 30 cm apart in the centre of the trench. Once they are established, feed them weekly with a weak solution of liquid fertilizer. Celery needs plenty of water, so be careful not to let it dry out.

When the plants are about 30 cm high, it is time to start blanching. Place a 10 cm collar of newspaper around the bottom of the plants, then draw some of the earth from the ridges around the collar and firm well. Repeat this each week until only a small tuft of leaves remain. It is also advisable to sprinkle some salt around to deter slugs from eating the celery. The heads will need protecting in severe weather conditions.

Blanching usually takes 6-8 weeks, after which time the celery should be mature enough to begin harvesting. Dig up sufficient heads for immediate use, leaving the remainder until required.

Part used: Stalks, leaves and roots.

Preparation: Remove all leaves, trim off the roots and wash thoroughly to remove dirt. Use the thicker outer branches for dicing and cooking, and the inner branches and leaves in salads. Celery is an ingredient in many soups. However, nutritionally, it is better to eat celery raw to preserve its medicinal properties.

Chickpeas – *Cicer arietinum*

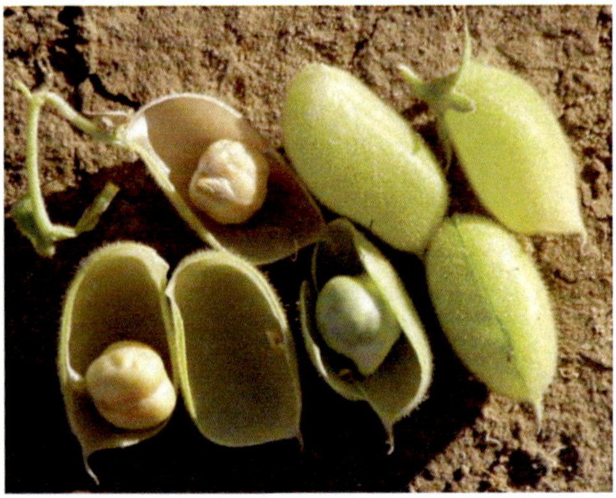

Chickpeas grow best in a subtropical or tropical climate with an average annual rainfall of 40 cm or above. Although they can be grown in a more moderate climate, yields will be much lower.

Properties and medicinal uses: Chickpeas are a valuable source of protein, zinc and folate. Being also very high in dietary fibre (and hence a healthy source of carbohydrates) they are ideal for anyone with insulin sensitivity or diabetes. Chickpeas are also a low-fat vegetable, most of which is polyunsaturated.

Recent studies by government agencies have also shown that they can assist in the lowering of cholesterol in the bloodstream.

Planting time and harvesting: ***Sprouted chickpeas.*** Place the chickpeas in a clean jam jar; put a piece of netting or muslin over the top of the jar and secure in place (this will act as a sieve); water overnight or for at least 8 hours. Next day, sieve the water by inverting the jar, rinse the sprouts and replace with fresh water. In warm weather, rinse your sprouts twice daily, as they will become more easily dehydrated; in colder weather, once is usually enough. Be sure to drain well after each rinse. (It doesn't matter whether the jar is kept in light or shade at this stage, but direct sunlight is best avoided.)

Repeat this process every day for 4-5 days until the shoots begin sprouting. This is when you can start using them in salads on a daily basis. When your sprouts are ready they should be kept in an airtight container (their original jar will suffice) and kept in the fridge. This way further growth is inhibited and they will stay fresh for 3-4 days.

If you prefer, you can buy a ready-made container for sprouting; however, the method of sprouting remains the same.

Part used: Peas, sprouts.

Preparation: Chickpeas can be eaten cooked in stews or raw in salads (before or after they produce shoots). They can also be ground into flour called 'gram flour', 'chickpea flour' or 'besan' and used primarily in Indian cuisine. When ground and shaped into balls they can be fried as falafel or cooked and ground into a paste called hummus. Chick peas can be used in the making of curries and are one of the most popular vegetarian foods in the UK.

Chicory – *Cichorium intybus*

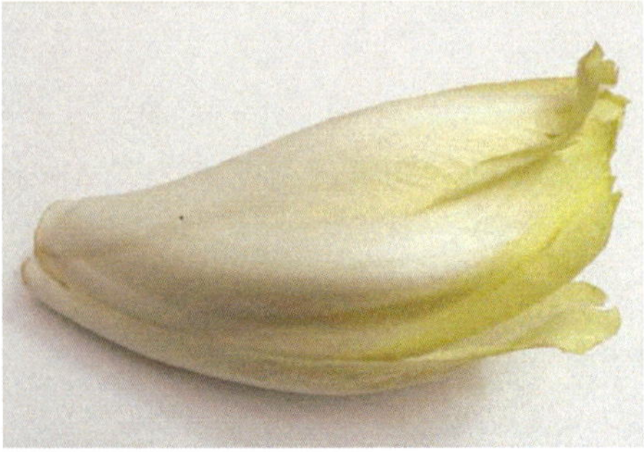

Copyright © 2007 David Monniaux

Chicory is grown for its leaves and usually eaten raw in salads, although it does have other culinary uses. Three types of cultivated chicory are generally grown: Radicchio, which has variegated red or red and green leaves – its taste is bitter and spicy but mellows when cooked; Sugarloaf, which looks similar to cos lettuce; and Belgian endive (or chicory in the UK), which has a small head of cream-coloured, bitter leaves and is grown completely underground or indoors in the absence of sunlight.

Properties and medicinal uses: Chicory is well known for its toxicity to internal parasites. It can also be used as a tonic, a treatment for gallstones, gastro-enteritis, sinus problems and cuts and bruises.

Planting time and harvesting: Chicory grows well in any soil, provided it is not in heavy shade. The seeds should be sown thinly in drills approximately 30-37.5 cm apart. The drills should be no deeper than 13 mm. Sprinkle the seed thinly along the drill and cover lightly with soil.

When large enough to handle, thin out the seedlings to 15 cm apart, water well and hoe around the plants regularly during the growing season.

Harvest the chicory in October or November when the leaves start to turn yellow, but definitely before the frosts begin. Lift the roots, twist off the leaves and snap off the thin root end, leaving a plump, stubby root 20 cm or so in length.

These roots should be packed the right way up in sand, soil or well-firmed peat in deep boxes/large pots.

Place in a warm cellar or warm, dark, frost-free shed, then cover with another box or pot, to eliminate light. The chicory will be ready for eating in about 3-4 weeks.

Part used: The whole chicory.

Preparation: Wash well. Cut the chicory in half before cooking. The leaves can be stuffed, baked, boiled, cut and cooked, or eaten raw in salad.

China rose radish sprouts – *Raphanus sativus*

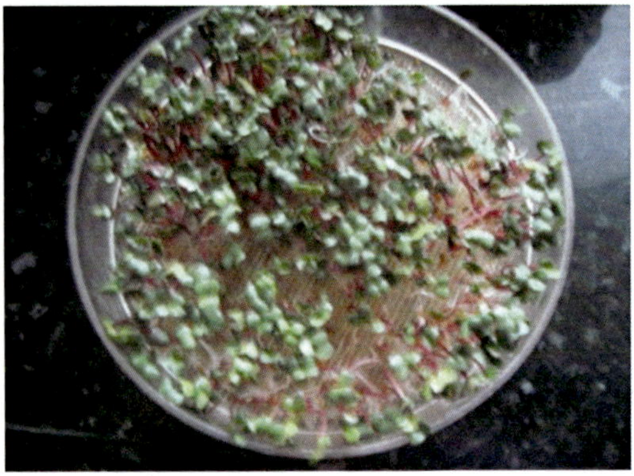

China rose radish is conspicuous by its long, tapered roots comprising red skin and white, crisp flesh.

Properties and medicinal uses: China rose radish is very high in vitamin C, while the diuretic effect of radish sprouts help to cleanse the digestive tract. It is also good for easing coughs, soothing sore throats, clearing sinuses and reducing fever.

Planting time and harvesting: ***Sprouted china rose radish.*** Place the china rose radish seeds in a clean jam jar; put a piece of netting or muslin over the top of the jar and secure in place (this will act as a sieve); water overnight or for at least 8 hours. Next day, sieve the water by inverting the jar, rinse the sprouts and replace with fresh water. In warm weather, rinse your sprouts twice daily, as they will become more easily dehydrated; in colder weather, once is usually enough. Be sure to drain well after each rinse. (It doesn't matter whether the jar is kept in light or shade at this stage, but direct sunlight is best avoided.)

Repeat this process every day for 4-5 days until the shoots begin sprouting. This is when you can start using them in salads on a daily basis. When your sprouts are ready they should be kept in an airtight container (their original jar will suffice) and kept in the fridge. This way further growth is inhibited and they will stay fresh for 3-4 days.

If you would prefer, you can buy a ready-made container for sprouting; however, the method of sprouting remains the same.

Part used: Roots, sprouts.

Preparation: Eaten raw in salads before or after they produce the shoots or can be mixed in juice for their nutritious benefits.

China rose radish has a spicy, hot flavour and is good mixed with milder varieties of sprouts in salads and sandwiches, or on their own with any meal for a stronger taste.

Courgettes - *Cucurbita pepo*

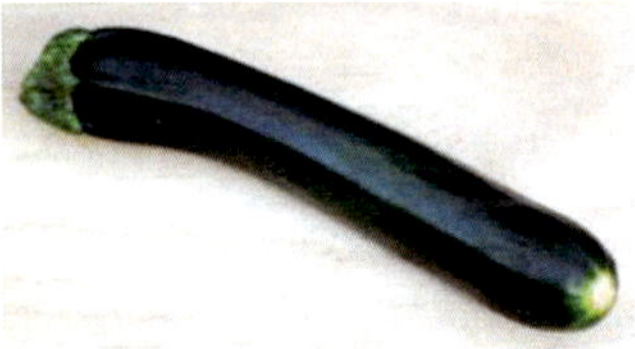

The courgette is a popularly cultivated summer squash and is native to the Americas. It is a variety of *Cucurbit* and related to the cucumber, gherkin, squash and watermelon. It has a darkish green skin with firm pale flesh and is known in some countries as zucchini.

Properties and medicinal uses: The courgette contains folic acid, potassium and vitamin A. It is also a good source of vitamin C, which can help prevent conditions like scurvy, bruising etc, and lutein which promotes eye health. The high fibre content of the courgette can help protect against colon cancer.

When cooking and eating courgettes, do not remove the skin as it contains beta-carotene, a vitamin that acts as an antioxidant and protects cells against oxidation damage.

The courgette has a high water content and contains just 25 calories (or approximately 15 calories per 100g). This makes it an ideal vegetable for those wishing to lose weight.

Planting time and harvesting: The seeds should be sown between March and the end of May. Fill a 7.5 cm pot with compost and firm down gently. Sow a seed vertically 2.5 cm deep and cover lightly with more compost. Label the pot, water the soil and place in a propagator or on a windowsill. When roots show through the bottom of the pot, transfer to a 12.5 cm container.

Transplant the seedlings into the garden in late spring/early summer. Ensure the soil is well dug, well-drained and rich in nutrients. The courgette will thrive in a sunny location, protected from harsh winds.

It is essential to give the plants plenty of water, particularly when they are in flower and when the fruits start to swell. Mulch the area well to lock in moisture. In heavy, well-manured soil, the plants will not require any additional feed; however, in a light or sandy soil, spray them regularly with a good liquid feed.

Harvest the courgettes as required when they are roughly 10 cm long. If harvested 2-3 times a week, it will help keep the plants productive throughout the season.

Part used: Fruit.

Preparation: Wash the courgettes well but do not peel them. Cut off the stem and slice the fruit. Boil them in a little slightly salted water for approximately 10 minutes. Serve hot, seasoned with salt, pepper and olive oil.

Courgettes can also be eaten baked, grilled or grated raw over salad.

Cucumber – *Cucumis sativus*

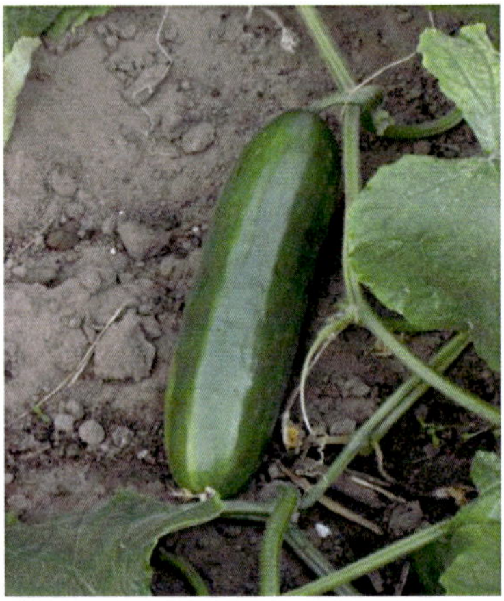

Copyright © 2005 Rasbak

The cucumber is member of the gourd family. The plant is a creeping vine that roots in the earth and grows up a supporting frame. It has large leaves that cover and protect the fruit. Originally native to India, it is now grown in many countries around the world.

Properties and medicinal uses: The cucumber is an excellent source of vitamin C and folic acid, while the fibre in its skin contains potassium, magnesium and silica. A few of its innumerable health benefits are listed below:

- the removal of waste and toxins built up in the body
- cucumber and carrot juice can ease rheumatic conditions caused by excessive uric acid
- an aid in the control of diabetes

- helps those suffering from chest, lung and stomach problems
- its potassium helps regulate blood pressure and promote flexibility of the muscles
- its magnesium aids efficient blood circulation and relaxes nerves and muscles
- fresh cucumber juice reduces heartburn, soothes acid stomach and gastritis
- its silica contributes to the strength of the body's connective tissue.

Planting time and harvesting: Sow each cucumber seed individually, on its edge, in a 7.5 cm pot containing rich soil. Begin sowings for greenhouse cultivation in January and continue through to late April, at reasonable intervals. Water in, and keep the air moist and well-ventilated.

For indoor cucumbers, replant them in their growing beds when they are approximately 15 cm tall; as they grow you will need to tie them to a frame for support. When established, loosely tie a loop of soft, strong string around the stem of the plants, and attach the other end to the top wire. The plant stem will gradually curl up and around this string as it grows. The growing point should be pinched when it reaches the top of the frame. Pinch out the tip of each side shoot at 2 leaves beyond a female flower (female flowers have a miniature cucumber behind them, while male flowers have just a thin stalk). Pinch out tips of flowerless side shoots when they are 120 cm long. Feed every 2 weeks with a tomato fertilizer once the first fruits have started to swell.

Harvest each fruit as and when it is ready; this promotes further development. Fresh cucumbers are firm and bright green in colour. If dark green or yellowish, they are past their best.

Part used: The whole fruit.

Preparation: Wash thoroughly. If served raw there is no need to peel the cucumber unless the skin is very tough. Drink as a juice, eat fresh in salads or in finger-size chunks in dips.

Dandelion – *Taraxacum officinale*

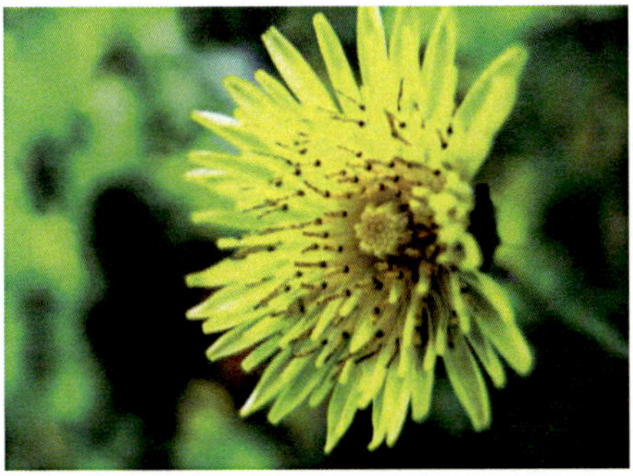

The dandelion is a biennial or perennial herbaceous plant, which is taprooted (it has a large, single root that grows vertically downwards and bears smaller lateral roots). Its leaves are approximately 5-25 cm long and form a crown below the flower, which is golden yellow in colour.

All too common in most gardens, the dandelion is often thought of as a weed to be destroyed at all costs. However, it is actually beneficial and has a wide range of uses.

Properties and medicinal uses: Dandelion leaves are rich in vitamins and minerals, especially vitamins A, C and K, and a good source of calcium, potassium, iron and manganese. The dandelion is regularly used by Medical Herbalists to treat a variety of disorders such as infections, bile and liver problems, and as a diuretic. It is a traditional old remedy and is shown to have anti-inflammatory effects and assist with urinary tract infections in women.

Planting time and harvesting: Seeds should be sown in April and the resulting plants thinned to 15 cm apart. Harvest the roots in

October. If the leaves are to be used in salads, cover the crowns with boxes in the following spring to produce balanced leaves. Dandelion leaves should be fairly large and have a fresh, green appearance.

Part used: Leaves and root.

Preparation: Wash the leaves well. Scrub the roots and trim off any rootlets. The leaves can be eaten raw in salads or used as a green vegetable. The flower petals make an acceptable dandelion wine, while the roasted, ground roots can be used as a caffeine-free coffee substitute. The leaves are cooked in the same way as cabbage greens. The roots should be roasted until thoroughly dried and shrivelled.

Fennel – *Foeniculum vulgare var. azoricum*

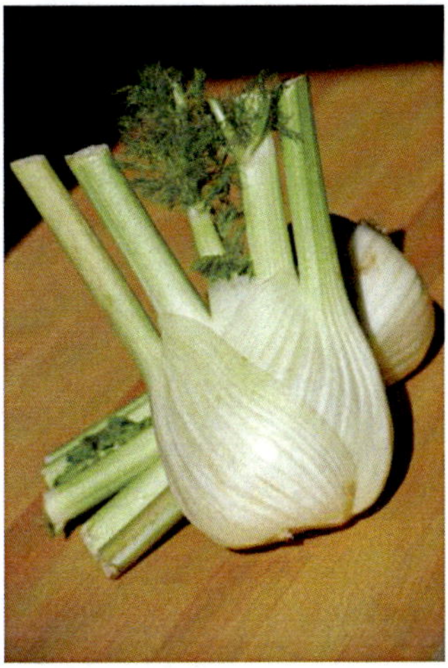

Copyright © 2008 Rolf Krahl (Rotkraut)

There are two varieties of fennel normally grown. The first variety is the common fennel, which is a perennial herb. The second, Florence fennel, or finocchio (its Italian name), has similar leaves but is grown for its bulbous stem. It is with this second variety that we are concerned here.

Properties and medicinal uses: Fennel contains anethole and, due to its carminative properties, is chiefly used in purgatives to alleviate their side effects.

Fennel water can help increase breast milk in nursing mothers. Fennel made into a syrup can be used to treat babies with colic.

For adults, fennel seeds or tea can relax the intestines and reduce bloating caused by digestive disorders. You can make fennel tea by pouring boiling water on a teaspoonful of bruised fennel seeds.

Planting time and harvesting: In May, sow the seeds in 15 cm pots and thin out to 1-2 seedlings per pot until mid-June. Then plant out at 25 cm apart in rich loam (soil that contains about 60% sand, 30% silt and 20% clay), in a sunny location. Keep the area weed free and as the leaf bases begin to swell, draw the soil up around them to blanch them (keep them white).

Harvest the fennel in late August when well developed and tender, lifting as required.

Part used: Bulb, leaves, seeds.

Preparation: Wash well. Scrape the bulbs and cut both the bulbs and stalk into 2.5 cm slices and braise in a little milk until tender. The bulb may also be sautéed, stewed or grilled but do not overcook as the strong aniseed flavour is reduced by cooking.

The bulb, foliage and seeds of the fennel plant are also commonly eaten raw in salads. Dried fennel seeds are brown or green in colour when fresh but slowly turn a dull grey as they age. For cooking and salads, green seeds are best. The leaves have a subtle flavour and are similar in shape to dill.

Garlic – *Allium sativum*

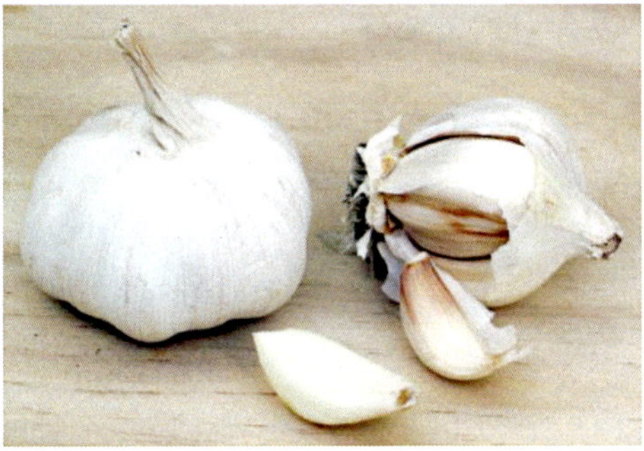

Copyright © 2005 Donovan Govan

Garlic is native to Central Asia and is member of the onion family (*Alliaceae*), along with the shallot, leek and chive. Its bulb contains up to 20 fleshy sections called cloves, which can be eaten either raw or cooked, or used for medicinal purposes.

Properties and medicinal uses: When garlic is crushed it yields allicin, a compound that exhibits antibiotic and antifungal properties, and which is believed to help speed up recovery from minor ailments.

Studies have shown that matured garlic can have a strong antioxidant effect that helps protect the body against harmful 'free radicals'.

It has been found that countries where garlic is consumed in higher amounts have a lower prevalence of cancer.

Planting time and harvesting: The cloves are planted in mid-October and harvested in late spring. Plant the individual cloves outdoors directly into a rich, light soil that will not become waterlogged over winter. Plant each clove in an upright position (with the pointed end facing up) 2.5 cm below the soil surface. Space each clove about 10cm apart, in rows roughly 45 cm apart.

To harvest, ease the bulbs out of the soil when the leaves are down and have lost their greenness. Set them aside and let them to dry in the sun for a few days but take them indoors if there is rain about. When they are dry, hang them up in a net bag or plait them into a string and store where it is cool and airy.

Part used: Bulb.

Preparation: Garlic is best eaten raw in salad but may be applied to breads to create a variety of dishes, e.g. garlic bread/garlic toast. Separate the bulb into cloves and coat them by dribbling olive oil (or any other oil-based seasoning) over them. Roast in an oven.

Garlic has a strong flavour that mellows and sweetens significantly when cooked. It can be used in stir-fries with eggs, meat and vegetables, or braised like asparagus.

Horseradish – *Armoracia rusticana*

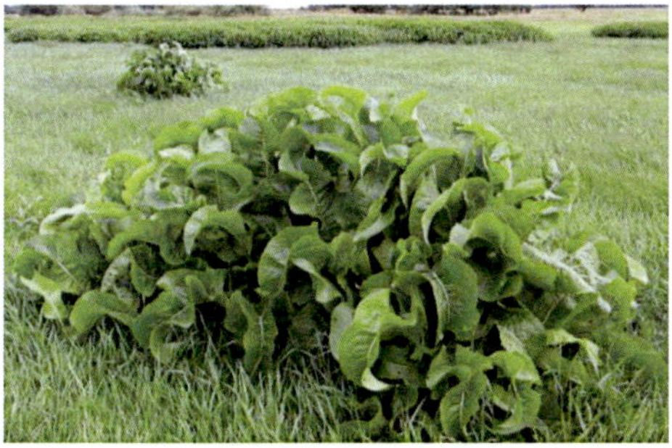

Copyright © 2009 Christian Fischer

Horseradish is a perennial plant of the Brassicaceae family, which includes mustard, broccoli and cabbages. It grows up to 1.5 metres tall and produces white flowers in the spring. It is mainly grown for its large white, tapered root.

Properties and medicinal uses: Horseradish contains vitamin C, potassium, calcium, magnesium and phosphorus, plus volatile oils, such as mustard oil, which has antibacterial properties. Its roots have been used to treat a variety of minor health problems, including urinary tract infections, bronchitis, sinus congestion and coughs.

Planting time and harvesting: Take root cuttings in early spring. Select 15 cm long pieces of root about 2.5 cm thick. Plant them in the garden directly into the soil at a depth of 5 cm and space them about 30 cm apart. Maintain the soil well as any cuttings will take about three years to grow to maturity. Horseradish will grow best in a light, well-dug, rich, moist soil.

Spray the horseradish plants with a general purpose liquid fertilizer about once a fortnight during summer. When the roots are mature (3 years old) dig them up and store them in sand in a dark, frost-free place for the winter.

Part used: Root, greens.

Preparation: Wash the root but do not cook it as it will lose its nutritional properties. We usually think of 'horseradish' as the ready-prepared grated root of the horseradish plant mixed with vinegar. Thus prepared, it is a white to creamy-beige colour. While it will happily keep for many months in the fridge, it will eventually start to darken, which means it's ready to be replaced. The leaves of the plant ('horseradish greens') are also edible but are not commonly eaten.

Horseradish sauce is usually served with roast beef but can be used in a number of other dishes, e.g. sandwiches or salads, or as a main ingredient for soups.

Kale (borecole) – *Brassica oleracea*

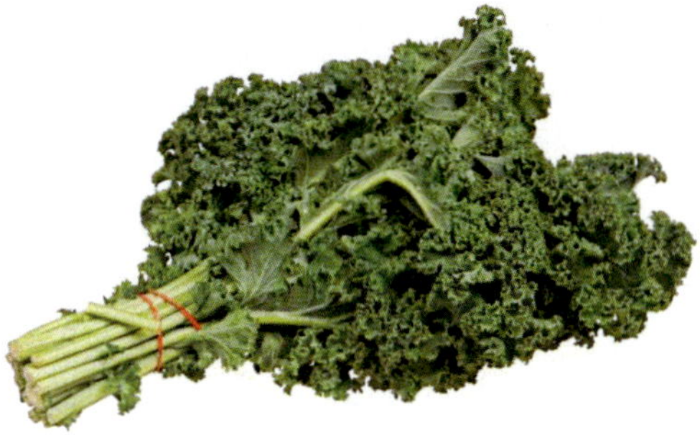

Kale is a form of cabbage (the *Brassica oleracea Acephala* Group, which also includes broccoli, cauliflower, brussels sprouts and collard greens).

Properties and medicinal uses: Kale is very nutritious and has powerful antioxidant and anti-inflammatory properties. It is also very high in beta carotene, vitamin K, vitamin C, lutein, zeaxanthin, and quite rich in calcium.

Kale contains sulforaphane (especially if chopped or minced), a chemical believed to have potent anti-cancer properties. Boiling the kale will result in a decrease in the level of its anti-cancer compounds, whilst steaming, microwaving and stir frying results in only a minor loss. Kale also contains indole-3-carbinol, a chemical that boosts DNA repair.

Planting time and harvesting: Kale is a winter vegetable and is cultivated as the cabbage and greens. Choose kale that is dark green in colour. Leaves with a slight brown tinge at the edges can be trimmed for use.

Part used: Curly leaves.

Preparation: Cut off any roots or stalk and wash thoroughly. Remove any hard, coarse ribs from the leaves and trim away brown edges. Kale freezes well and actually tastes better after being exposed to frost.

Kale greens are ideal in salads, particularly when combined with other strongly flavoured ingredients as dry-roasted peanuts, roasted almonds or red pepper flakes.

Kale can also be mixed with mashed potatoes or used in stir-fries.

Leeks – *Allium ampeloprasum var porrum*

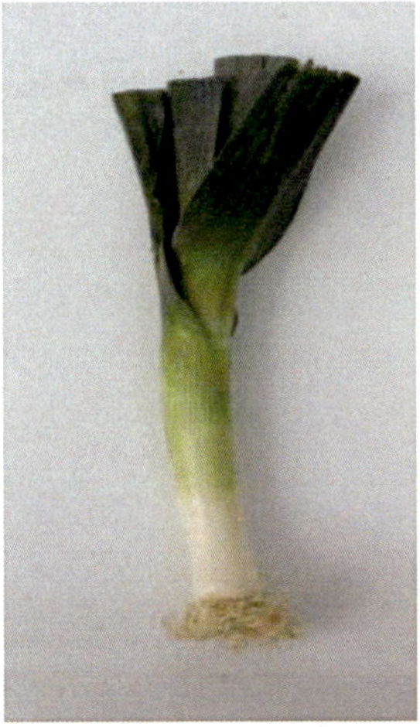

The leek is a member of the *Alliaceae* allium family, along with onions and garlic. Thought to be native to central Asia, they have been cultivated both there and across Europe throughout antiquity. Unlike the onion, the leek does not produce a tight bulb but forms a long roll of leaf sheaths.

Properties and medicinal uses: Leeks contain an impressive amount of polyphenols, including the flavonoid *kaempferol*, believed to reduce the risk of cancer. The substantial quantity of sulphur found in leeks supports the body's antioxidant system and the formation of connective tissue. Leeks are an excellent source of manganese, calcium, potassium, vitamin C, iron, folic acid, and vitamin B6. They also have laxative, antiseptic, diuretic, and anti-arthritic properties.

Planting time and harvesting: Leeks are best grown on moist, light, heavily manured soil. Prepare a nursery seed bed and sow the leeks in late March/early April for harvesting from September-April the following year. Make the drills 13 mm deep, 15 cm apart. Sow the leek seeds thinly, and at an early stage of development thin them out to 5 cm apart.

The seedlings can be transplanted to their main growing bed in June or July when they reach approximately 15-20 cm high. When lifting the seedlings out of the nursery bed, soak the soil first and lift them carefully using a hand fork. Lop off the top quarter of the leaves with scissors.

Transplant the seedlings into the main growing bed in holes 15 cm deep and 23 cm apart, in rows 38 cm apart. Drop them into the holes leaving just the tips of the leaves showing (planting them deeply helps to blanch the stems). Do not fill in the holes or cover the roots with soil. Fill each hole with water – this will wash some soil over the roots and be just enough to secure the plants. The holes will fill up naturally from hoeing or rain. In time, when the holes have filled up, push some soil up to the stems using the hoe; this will encourage a good length of white (blanched) stem. This should be done gradually over a 3-week period – if done too soon the plants are likely to rot.

Leeks are an extremely hardy vegetable and can be left in the ground throughout autumn and winter. Harvest when required.

Part used: Stem or stalk.

Preparation: Remove the outer layer and wash well. Chop into slices 5-10 mm thick. Leeks are often used to flavour soup. Boiling makes it soft and milder in taste; frying leaves it crunchier and preserves the taste; it can also be eaten raw in salads.

Lentils – *Lens culinaris*

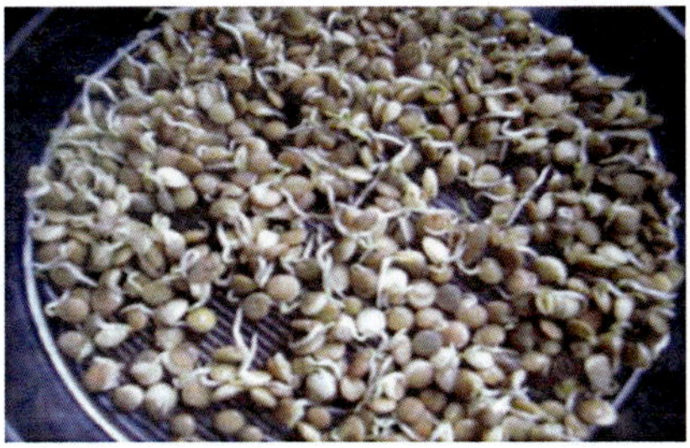

Lentils grow in pods on a bushy annual plant of the *Legume* family. The plant is believed to have originated in the Near East and has been part of the human diet since Neolithic times. Their colours range from yellow to a reddish-orange to green, brown and black.

Properties and medicinal uses: Lentils contain high levels of proteins, including the essential amino acids isoleucine and lysine. Although lentils are deficient in two essential amino acids, methionine and cysteine, sprouted lentils contain sufficient levels of all essential amino acids, including methionine and cysteine. Lentils also contain dietary fibre, folic acid, vitamin B1 and minerals. Lentils are also a good source of iron, making them useful for preventing iron deficiency in adolescents, pregnant women and those with Coeliac disease.

However, lentils do contain trypsin inhibitors and a fairly high phytate content. Trypsin is an enzyme involved in digestion and phytates reduce the bioavailability of dietary minerals. Phytates can be reduced by soaking the lentils in warm water overnight.

Planting time and harvesting: ***Sprouted lentils.*** Place the lentil seeds in a clean jam jar; put a piece of netting or muslin over the top of the jar and secure in place (this will act as a sieve); water overnight or for at least 8 hours. Next day, sieve the water by inverting the jar, rinse the sprouts and replace with fresh water. In warm weather, rinse your sprouts twice daily, as they will become more easily dehydrated; in colder weather, once is usually enough. Be sure to drain well after each rinse. (It doesn't matter whether the jar is kept in light or shade at this stage, but direct sunlight is best avoided.)

Repeat this process every day for 4-5 days until the shoots begin sprouting. This is when you can start using them in salads on a daily basis. When your sprouts are ready they should be kept in an airtight container (their original jar will suffice) and kept in the fridge. This way further growth is inhibited and they will stay fresh for 3-4 days.

If you would prefer, you can buy a ready-made container for sprouting; however, the method of sprouting remains the same.

Part used: Seeds.

Preparation: Lentils should never be eaten raw, due to the presence of phytic acid and tannins; some types of lentils require soaking overnight before cooking as well. Lentils require a cooking time of 10-30 minutes, depending on the variety. Lentils can be used as an inexpensive, nutritious ingredient in soup. Dried lentils can also be sprouted, as shown above, by leaving in water for several hours or overnight. This changes their nutrition profile.

Lettuce – *Lactuca sativa*

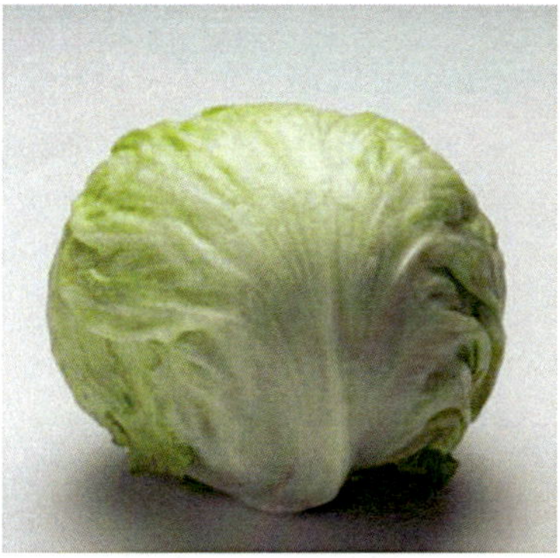

Copyright © 2006 Yorvik

Lettuce is an annual or biennial plant of the daisy family *Asteraceae* and originates from the Mediterranean. There are many varieties of lettuce, e.g. those with smaller or larger leaves, more loosely or tightly packed leaves, leaves that range from light green to deep, dark red, and different flavoured leaves.

Properties and medicinal uses: Lettuce is very low in calories and a source of vitamin A and folic acid. In ancient Rome and Egypt people would end a meal by eating lettuce to induce sleep, as all varieties contain lactucarium, a mild opiate-like substance.

High in dietary fibre, lettuce aids digestion. It has been associated with reducing the risk of cancer, heart disease, stroke and cataracts, due to its beta-carotene content, and linked with better liver health, being helpful in treating constipation, acid indigestion, arthritis, catarrh, circulatory problems. The juice of lettuce mixed with rose oil and applied to the forehead can help ease headaches and promote a sound night's sleep.

Planting time and harvesting: Lettuce does not thrive well after being moved, so sow seeds directly into a growing bed of rich soil. Scatter the seeds very thinly into drills 13 mm deep, in rows 30 cm apart. Water in the morning or at noon, but not in the evening, as that is more likely to encourage disease. When the seedlings produce their first leaves, thin them out to 15 cm-30 cm apart depending on the variety (do not overcrowd the bed).

Lettuce is a quick growing vegetable and therefore a good cash crop, which can be sown in between slower growing vegetables such as parsnips.

Part used: Leaf, stem.

Preparation: Remove roots and outer leaves. Separate remaining leaves and wash thoroughly. Lettuce leaves can be used whole or shredded, eaten raw in salads or cooked, as in Chinese cuisine when the stem is used along with the leaf.

Mung beans – *Vigna radiata*

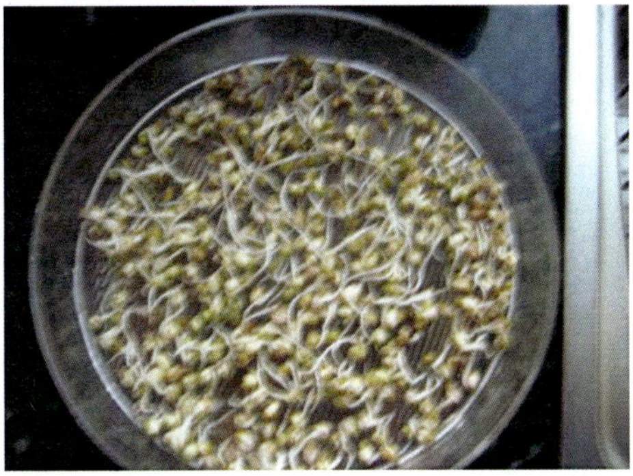

The mung bean is native to Bangladesh, India and Pakistan. The beans are small, ovoid, and green in colour.

Properties and medicinal uses: Mung bean sprouts contain rich quantities of vitamins A, B, C and E. They are also an excellent source of minerals, e.g. calcium, iron and potassium. The mung bean is an ideal food for weight watchers, as it has a very low fat content. A rich source of protein and fibre, it can also help lower high cholesterol. The complex carbohydrates in the mung bean aids digestion. They also help stabilize blood sugar and prevent its rapid rise at the end of a meal. Sufferers of diabetes or high cholesterol are recommended frequent consumption of mung beans. In Chinese medicine, mung bean sprouts are believed to contain anti-cancer properties. They also use them as a coolant for hot, inflammatory conditions.

Planting time and harvesting: ***Sprouted mung beans.*** Place the beans in a clean jam jar; put a piece of netting or muslin over the top of the jar and secure in place (this will act as a sieve); water overnight or for at least 8 hours. Next day, sieve the water by inverting the jar, rinse the sprouts and replace with fresh water. In warm weather, rinse your sprouts twice daily, as they will become more easily dehydrated; in colder weather, once is usually enough. Be sure to drain well after each rinse. (It doesn't matter whether the jar is kept in light or shade at this stage, but direct sunlight is best avoided.)

Repeat this process every day for 4-5 days until the shoots begin sprouting. This is when you can start using them in salads on a daily basis. When your sprouts are ready they should be kept in an airtight container (their original jar will suffice) and kept in the fridge. This way further growth is inhibited and they will stay fresh for 3-4 days.

If you would prefer, you can buy a ready-made container for sprouting; however, the method of sprouting remains the same.

Part used: Seeds.

Preparation: Generally eaten either whole (with or without skins) or as bean sprouts. Whole mung beans are generally prepared from dried beans by boiling until they are soft.

Mung bean sprouts can be stir-fried as a vegetable accompaniment to a meal, usually with ingredients such as garlic, ginger and spring onions. They can also be eaten in soup but to retain the nutrients of the beans they are best eaten in salads.

Onion (red) – *Allium cepa*

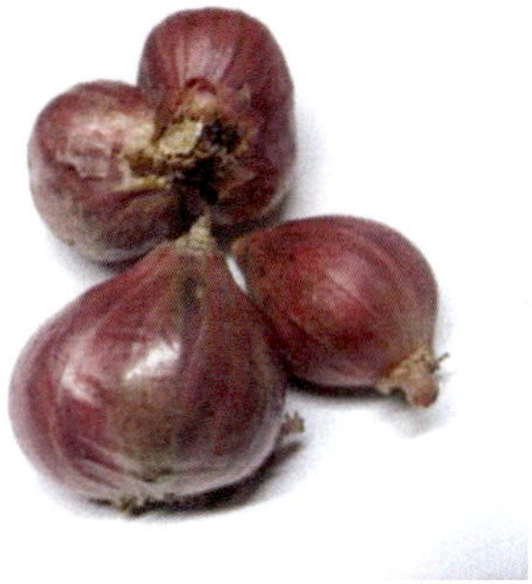

Copyright © 2003 Caduser

Red onions are cultivars of the onion with purplish-red skin and white flesh tinged with red. They are usually medium to large in size and have a mild, sweet flavour. Their colour comes from anthocyanidins such as cyanidin. Red onions are high in flavonoids. They can be stored for 3-4 months at room temperature.

Properties and medicinal uses: The more red onion you consume, the lower your blood-sugar glucose levels will be. This is due to the allyl propyl disulphide and chromium found in red onions. The chromium and vitamin B6 found in onions lower blood pressure and cholesterol, helping to increase cardiovascular health. And if you hope to lower your chances of colon cancer and related diseases, include red onions in your diet at least twice a week. Quercitin, one of the flavonoids found in onions, is known to be very beneficial to the health of the gastrointestinal tract. Red onions have also been shown to be beneficial to bone health. A compound known as GPCS inhibits cells that break down bones. Red onions can also reduce inflammation in the bones and throat, as well as in blood vessels. This reduces many of the symptoms of osteoporosis, asthma and even the common cold.

Planting time and harvesting: Red onions are easy to grow, frost-tolerant and like cool, wet spring weather. They prefer rich, well-drained soil with a pH of 6.2 to 6.8 (add lime if necessary). Grow red onions in raised beds about 10 cm high and 50 cm wide, with compost worked into the soil. Water consistently and keep weed-free while onions are maturing.

Plant onion sets 2-4 weeks before the last frost and use bulbs that are less than 2 cm in diameter. Onion sets should be spaced from 10-15 cm apart, depending on the size of the mature bulb. Press bulbs gently into the soil about 2.5 cm deep with their pointed tips just breaking the surface.

If planting onions from seed, wait until the soil temperature is 10°C. Sow seeds 6.25 mm deep, 13 mm apart, with 30-45 cm between each row.

Part used: Bulb.

Preparation: Peel the onion and the outer skin will simply slip off. Red onions can be eaten raw, grilled or lightly cooked with other foods, or added as colour to salads. They tend to lose their redness when cooked. Once cut you must consume quickly as onion has the tendency to absorb environmental viruses and bacteria. Dispose of any leftover onion.

Parsnip – *Pastinaca sativa*

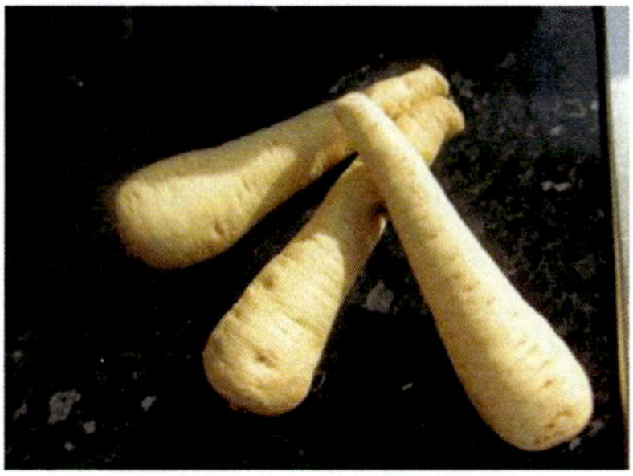

The parsnip is a root vegetable related to the carrot and originated in the Mediterranean area. It is paler and sweeter than the carrot, especially when cooked.

Properties and medicinal uses: Parsnips contain more vitamins and minerals than carrots, being an excellent source of vitamins B6, C, and E, fibre, folic acid, pantothenic acid, copper, manganese, niacin, thiamin, magnesium and potassium.

Planting time and harvesting: Parsnips are usually sown in late February or early March, to be ready for use from late October. Plant the seeds in groups of three or four, 13 mm deep and 12.5-15 cm apart, with rows 45 cm apart. Rake the soil over the drills lightly to cover the seeds. When the seedlings are big enough to be handled, thin them out to one at each station. Do not let the soil dry out completely (water in very dry conditions) and hoe regularly between the parsnips to keep the weeds down.

Parsnips can be harvested as required from October onwards and being a hardy crop can be left in the ground throughout winter. However, it is a good idea to lift a stock of roots to store in peat or sand in a cool place for use when the ground is frozen. Any roots still in the ground in early spring must be lifted before they start second growth or they will run straight to seed.

Part used: Root.

Preparation: Allow two medium sized roots for each serving. The roots should be smooth, firm and a good tapering shape. Wash, scrape or peel the roots, remove the leaf crowns and any rootlets. Parsnips can be boiled, steamed or roasted and served whole, in halves, quarters, slices or diced.

Peas (green) – *Pisum sativum*

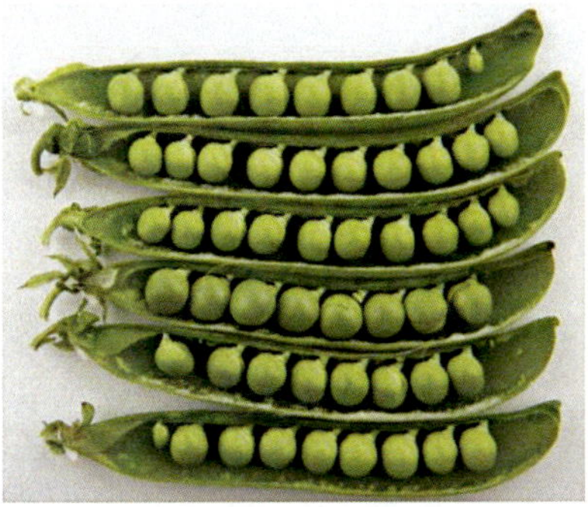

Copyright © 2011 Bill Ebeson

The pea is an annual plant with a life cycle of one year. It is a cool-season crop and is grown throughout the world. Although actually a fruit, the pea is used as a vegetable, and can be bought fresh, frozen, canned or dried.

Properties and medicinal uses: Peas are high in vitamins A, B, C, and lutein (a carotenoid that acts as an antioxidant and helps reduce the risk of age-related macular degeneration and cataracts). Being a low-calorie vegetable, peas are helpful as a weight-loss tool; and rich in dietary fibre, they are good for the relief of constipation.

Studies have shown that green peas could prove beneficial for lowering cholesterol levels, plus the high amount of iron and vitamin C they contain has been found to help strengthen the immune system.

Green peas slow down the appearance of glucose in the blood, thus helping to keep energy levels steady, aid nerve function and help maintain bone health.

The folic acid and vitamin B6 in green peas promote cardiovascular health, whilst being rich in antioxidants, like vitamin C, green peas can help keep cancer at bay.

Planting time and harvesting: The pea plant grows thin tendrils from leaves that coil around any available support and can climb to be 1-2 m high. One way to support climbing peas is to push branches pruned from trees or other woody plants upright into the soil, or use twine or netting supported by a frame. Pea plants are self-pollinating.

Planting can take place from winter to early summer depending on location. They should be grown outdoors during winter and not in greenhouses. Peas prefer a slightly acidic, well-drained soil.

Plant directly in the soil 4-6 weeks before the last frost or start plants indoors and transplant after the last frost. Plant seeds 13 mm deep, 3 cm apart in raised beds or 5 cm apart in a traditional garden. Rows should be 45 cm apart.

Pods should be harvested before they turn light green, when the peas fill up the pod. Pea pods do not keep well once picked, and if not used quickly are best preserved by drying, canning or freezing within a few hours of harvesting.

Part used: Pea seeds.

Preparation: Remove peas from pods and wash. Peas are usually boiled or steamed, which breaks down the cell walls and makes them taste sweeter and the nutrients more bio-available. While cooking, add some mint from the garden for flavouring. Fresh peas are also used in salads and casseroles. Pod peas (mange tout) can be added to stir-fries. Dried peas are often added to soup or simply eaten on their own.

Peppers (chilli) – *Capsicum annuum*

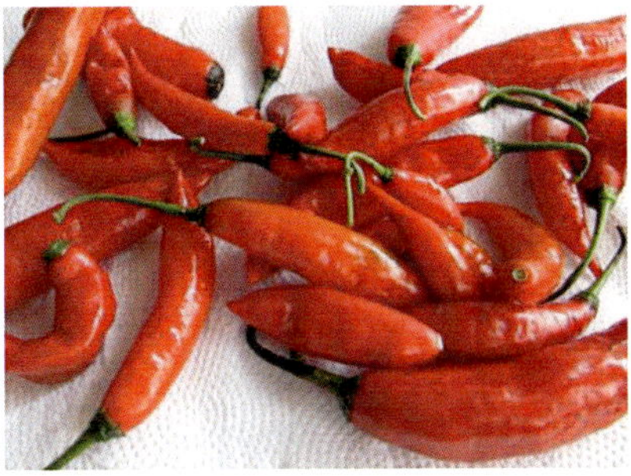

Chilli peppers are the fruit of plants from the genus *Capsicum* and are native to South and Central America, with India being the largest producer of chilli peppers in the world today.

Properties and medicinal uses: The substances that give chilli peppers their intensity when eaten or applied topically are capsaicin and several associated chemicals called *capsaicinoids*. When consumed, capsaicinoids trigger pain receptors in the mouth and throat to send a message to the brain that something hot has been eaten. The brain responds to this by raising the heart rate, increasing perspiration and the release of endorphins.

Capsaicin is also used as a safe and effective topical analgesic agent for the relief of arthritis pain, shingles pain, diabetic neuropathy, post-mastectomy pain and headaches.

Red chillies are a good source of vitamin C and carotene. Yellow and green chillies (which are the unripened fruit) contain significantly lower amounts of these substances. Peppers also contain most B vitamins, especially vitamin B6, and are very high in potassium, magnesium, and iron.

Planting time and harvesting: Sow the seeds in February/March, in a greenhouse or poly-tunnel, using soil-based compost for good drainage. Arrange 4-5 seeds *of the same variety* in 7.5 cm pots, at a depth of about 5 mm, cover with a little more compost, pat down gently, and lightly water the surface. Ensure they are kept warm, moist (but not wet) and well ventilated.

When the seedlings have about 5 pairs of leaves they should be potted on into 22.5 cm to 30 cm pots. In hot summers you may need to provide them with shade from the sun.

Once the fruits are well shaped, firm to the touch, with an even, glossy colour they can be harvested. The sooner you pick them, the more the plant will produce.

Part used: Pod.

Preparation: Chilli pepper pods can be used fresh or dried. Many fresh chillies have a tough outer skin which does not disintegrate in the cooking process. Where chillies are cooked whole or in large slices, the skin is usually charred or blistered to avoid completely cooking the flesh beneath. When cooled, the skins will slip off easily.

Fresh or dried chillies are often used to make hot chilli sauce, a condiment that adds spice to other dishes.

Peppers (sweet) – *Capsicum annuum*

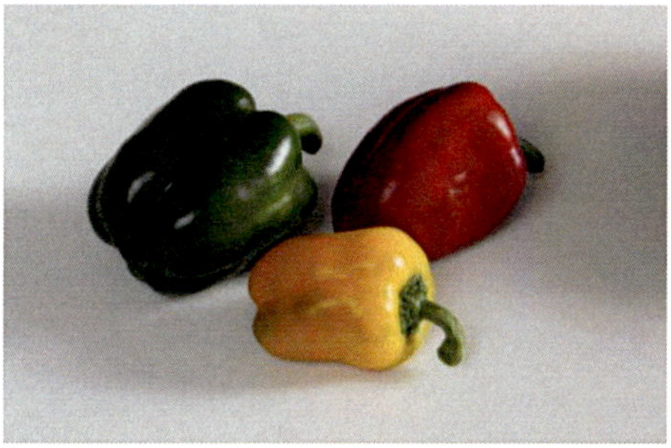

Copyright © 2009 Kham Tran

The sweet pepper is a cultivar group of the species *Capsicum annuum* (chilli pepper) and its plant produces fruits in different colours, including green, red, yellow and orange. Sweet peppers are native to Mexico, Central America and northern South America. The best fruit are those allowed to ripen fully on the plant in sunshine. Fruit harvested whilst still green and ripened in storage are not as sweet and tasty.

Properties and medicinal uses: Sweet peppers are crammed with nutrients. They are not only an excellent source of vitamin C, thiamin, vitamin B6, beta carotene and folic acid, but they also contain phytochemicals that have exceptional antioxidant activity. These phytochemicals include chlorogenic acid, zeaxanthin, and coumeric acid.

When assessing the nutrient values of the different coloured sweet peppers, it was noted that red peppers have significantly higher levels of valuable nutrients than green. Red peppers also contain lycopene, which is a carotene that helps protect against cancer and heart disease. They have also been shown to protect against cataracts, prevent blood clot formation and reduce the risk of heart attacks and strokes.

Planting time and harvesting: Sweet peppers are best grown from transplants. In late February/early March sow the seeds indoors, 2 per 7.5 cm pot, and thin the seedlings to one per pot when they are large enough to handle.

When the plants reach 15 cm-20 cm in height, transplant them into rich, well-dug cropping beds, allowing 0.3 sq m per plant. Water the plants regularly and a give them a light misting of water in the evening during flowering time.

Harvest green peppers when they have reached a useable size, but allow red peppers to mature and ripen on the plant before picking. Peppers should be well-shaped and firm to the touch, with an even, glossy colour.

Part used: The whole pepper

Preparation: Cut off the stem end and scoop out the seeds, then wash. Sweet peppers are frequently eaten chopped and raw in salads, or cooked in stir-fries. They can also be fried, roasted whole or in pieces, or chopped and used in salsas or other sauces.

Potato – *Solanum tuberosum*

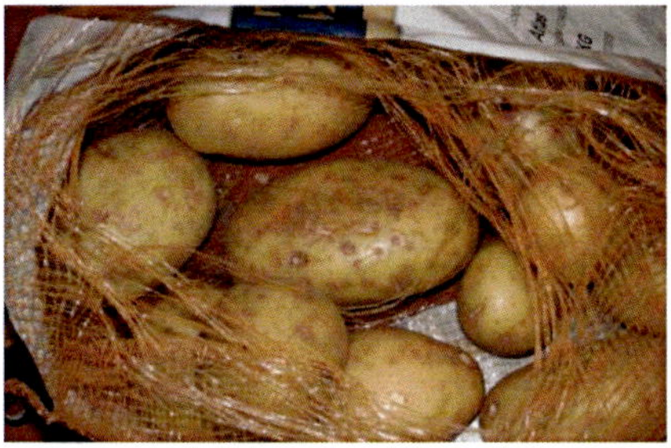

Copyright © 2011 Blonder1984

The potato is a perennial of the *Solanaceae* family and is native to Peru. The potato has white, brown, purple or red skin and white or golden flesh.

Properties and medicinal uses: The potato contains vitamin C, thiamin, niacin, vitamin B6, folic acid, pantothenic acid, iron, magnesium, potassium, copper and is packed with dietary fibre. The fibre in the potato provides bulk, which protects against colon cancer, improves glucose tolerance and insulin sensitivity, lowers plasma cholesterol and triglyceride concentrations and leaves one feeling fuller. Unfortunately, the potato is not considered as one of the daily recommended diet of five portions of fruit and vegetables.

Planting time and harvesting: In January, tray the seeds in a warm place prior to planting in late March/early April. Potatoes require rich, well-dug soil that was heavily manured the previous autumn. Before planting, incorporate a good, general fertiliser at roughly 100g per square meter. Plant the sets or seeds with a trowel 15 cm deep and 23 cm apart, with 60 cm between rows. As shoots emerge, draw the earth up, over and around them. Repeat this process as the growth increases until the potatoes are eventually growing on a ridge.

The potatoes can be harvested as soon as they are big enough, typically in June or early July. Late main crop potatoes should be harvested in October and stored for winter use by placing them in sacks or boxes in a dark, frost-free place.

Good quality potatoes are clean, firm and free from cracks and other surface defects. The skin on new potatoes is thin and rubs off easily. The skin thickens as the potatoes mature.

Any potato with green colouring on any of its surfaces should be avoided as they contain chlorophyll and are usually bitter.

Part used: Tuber.

Preparation: There are many ways to prepare potatoes, e.g. skin-on or peeled, whole or chopped, with or without seasoning. The only requirement involves cooking to swell the starch granules. Most potato dishes are served hot, but some are first cooked then served cold, for example potato salad and crisps.

Common dishes are: mashed potatoes, which are peeled, boiled for 10-25 minutes, then mashed with milk or yogurt and butter; whole baked potatoes; chips, sliced and fried (French fries); hash browns, grated into small thin strips and fried; Rösti, grated and formed into dumplings or pancakes.

Pumpkin – *Cucurbita pepo*

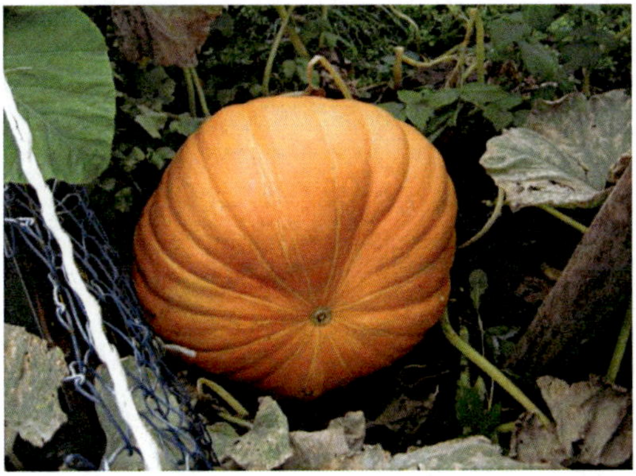

Copyright © 2009 Ude

The pumpkin is a squash of the *Cucurbitaceae* family and is native to North America. It has a thick, orange or yellow skin, which contains the seeds and pulp. The pumpkin has both male and female flowers on the same plant. The female flower is distinguished by the small ovary at the base of the petals. These bright and colourful flowers are extremely short-lived and may only open for one day.

Properties and medicinal uses: The medicinal properties of pumpkin are anti-diabetic, antioxidant, anti-carcinogenic and anti-inflammatory. It is low in fat and calories, and rich in nutrients such as alpha-carotene, beta-carotene, fibre, vitamins C and E, potassium, magnesium and pantothenic acid. Alpha-carotene and beta-carotene are powerful antioxidants and are pro-vitamin A carotenoids, which means that the body converts them to vitamin A. Beta-carotene may also reverse skin damage caused by high exposure to the sun. Alpha-carotene is also believed to slow the aging process, reduce the risk of developing cataracts and prevent growth of tumours. Carotenoids also boost the immune system and lessen the risk of heart disease.

Pumpkin seeds have numerous health benefits, being a good source of protein, magnesium, manganese, phosphorus, phytosterols, zinc, several vitamins, and are believed to lower cholesterol. Pumpkin seed oil contains essential fatty acids that help maintain healthy blood vessels, nerves and tissues.

Planting time and harvesting: In early spring, sow the seeds singly in 7.5 cm pots in a heated greenhouse, using good quality compost. The temperature should be a minimum of 21°C and the germination process should take 1-2 weeks. Soon after germination the seedlings will need re-potting into 12-15 cm pots, again with good potting compost.

In warmer parts of the country, and when there is no danger of further frosts, you can transplant the seedlings into the garden in late spring and protect with poly tunnels or glass cloches. However, being a warm weather crop, pumpkins are generally planted out in early July, in a sunny location. Ideally, the soil temperature at 7.5 cm deep should be at least 15.5° C and the soil should hold water well. Space out the seedlings to at least 90 cm apart (more if you have a larger garden). Mulch the surrounding area with well-rotted compost, repeating the mulch in mid-summer, and give plenty of water and nutrients at frequent intervals. Keep weeds under control.

Pinch out the growing tips when about two to four pumpkin fruits have formed; this will concentrate growth and control the size of the plant. To harvest, use a sharp knife to cut the ripe pumpkins, leaving about 7.5 cm of stem on the pumpkin.

Part used: Flesh, seeds, leaves, oil.

Preparation: Wash well, peel, remove the seeds, and dice the flesh. When ripe, pumpkins can be boiled, baked, steamed, roasted, made into a pie or included in soups. Pumpkin seeds are a popular snack that can be found hulled or semi-hulled at most grocery stores. Pumpkin seed oil is used in cooking or as a salad dressing.

Radish – *Raphanus sativus*

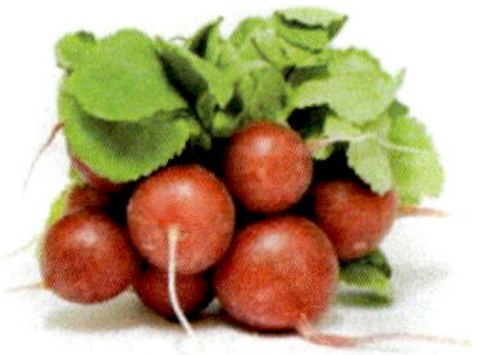

Radishes are edible roots of the *Brassicaceae* family. They can be categorized into four types (summer, autumn, winter and spring) and grow in a variety of shapes, colours, and sizes.

Properties and medicinal uses: Radishes are rich in ascorbic acid, folic acid and potassium. They are a good source of vitamin B6, riboflavin, magnesium, copper and calcium. They are also very good for the liver and the stomach and purify the blood, as well as being diuretic in nature, cleaning the kidneys and inhibiting infections in the kidneys and urinary systems.

Being a very good detoxifier and rich in vitamin C, folic acid and anthocyanins, radishes help cure many types of cancer, particularly those of colon, kidney, intestines, stomach and oral cancer. The vitamin C, phosphorus, zinc and vitamin B present in radishes, help to maintain the skin's natural moisture balance. Crushed raw radish is a refreshing cleanser and/or face pack. It also helps cure skin disorders, such as drying up, rashes, cracks etc.

Radishes have anti-pruritic properties that can be used as an effective treatment for insect bites and stings, reducing pain and swelling and soothing the affected area. They also relieve congestion of the respiratory system due to colds, infection and allergies.

Planting time and harvesting: Radish requires a sunny position in the garden, and to grow in sandy loam. Sow radish seeds directly into the ground at a depth of 1 cm, spacing them out to 2.5 cm between seeds, in rows 15 cm apart. Sowing the seeds close together helps to keep the resulting radishes smaller and tastier. As they grow, the seedlings are at the mercy of the flea beetle, which feed on the leaves; try sprinkling the seedlings with powdered dry soil if this is a problem.

Water the crop well, especially at the height of summer, and harvest the radishes when the roots are about the size of a 10 pence piece

Part used: Root, leaves, seeds.

Preparation: The most commonly eaten portion is the root although the entire plant is edible. The tops can be used as a leaf vegetable.

The root of the radish is usually eaten raw, although some hardier varieties can be steamed. The raw flesh has a crisp texture and a pungent, peppery flavour.

Radishes are used in salads, as well as in many European dishes.

Rhubarb – *Rheum rhabarbarum*

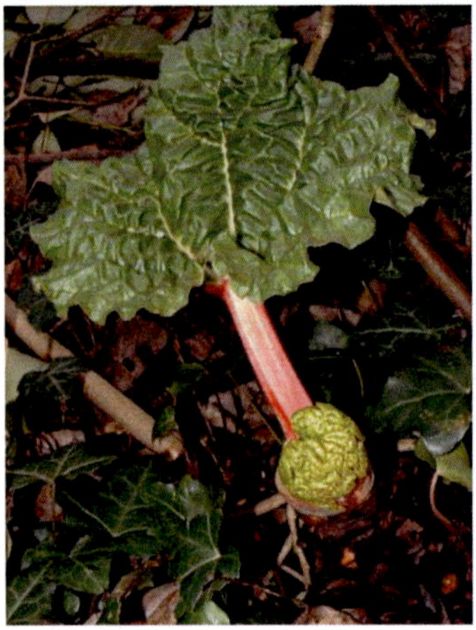

Copyright © 2008 Olivier

Rhubarb is a herbaceous perennial plant and native to Asia. Although eaten as a fruit, rhubarb is really a vegetable with a strong, tart flavour. Its leaves are toxic and should not be consumed.

Properties and medicinal uses: Roots and stems of the rhubarb are rich in anthraquinones, such as emodin and rhein and have been used as a strong laxative throughout antiquity. Rhubarb also has an astringent effect on the mucous membranes of the mouth and the nasal cavity.

Planting time and harvesting: Choose a partially shaded spot with free-draining soil and prepare the soil in advance by digging in lots of well-rotted organic matter. Rhubarb can be grown from seed but it is much quicker and simpler to grow them from one-year-old plants, known as 'crowns'. Crowns can be planted outside in late autumn/early winter. Despite their small size at this point, many varieties will grow very large, so ensure you leave at least 75 cm between them.

To plant, dig a hole a little wider than the plant and put in the crown ensuring that the top bud of each one is at, or just below, ground level. Firm down the soil and spread a mulch of compost over the top. Once the leaves have died back, spread on a new layer of compost to keep weeds in check and retain moisture. In spring, flowers will develop, so make sure you deadhead them as soon as they bud.

Harvest the rhubarb from May-June in their second growing season by picking the three largest stalks and gently twisting and pulling them from ground level. Do not harvest beyond late June, and leave at least three stems in place to allow the plants to recover for the following season. To keep your rhubarb healthy it should be divided every five or six years. Carry out this work in winter, splitting each plant into three or four crowns, and plant as you would for a young rhubarb.

Part used: Stalks.

Preparation: Wash thoroughly. Rhubarb can be dehydrated and mixed with fruit juice. In most cases, strawberry juice is used to mimic strawberry and rhubarb pie. Another method of cooking is to cut up the stalks into 2.5 cm pieces and stew them, (rhubarb stalks are very juicy, and so they only need the minimum of water to cover them). Then add ½ cup of Stevia granulated sugar for each pound of rhubarb, and cinnamon and/or nutmeg to taste. Boil the rhubarb until soft.

At this stage, cooked with strawberries or apples as a sweetener, or with stem or root ginger, rhubarb makes an excellent jam. Add the fruit at a ratio of two parts fruit to one part rhubarb. Continue boiling for at least ten minutes after fruit is completely softened.

Rhubarb can be stored in a plastic bag in the fridge for 2-3 weeks, frozen raw, or blanched for 1 minute in boiling water, or stewed to take up less space.

Spinach – *Spinacia oleracea*

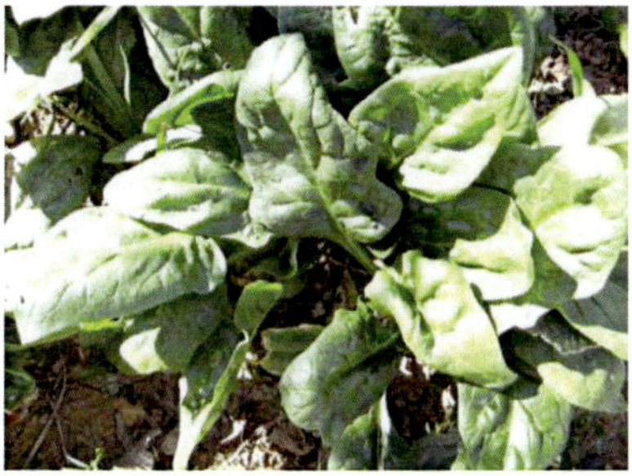

Spinach is an edible flowering plant native to Persia. It is an annual plant which grows to a height of up to 30 cm and may survive over winter in temperate regions. Fresh spinach loses a good deal of its nutritional value when stored for more than a few days. While refrigeration slows this effect to about eight days, spinach will lose most of its folic acid and carotenoid content. However, you can easily store spinach in the freezer for up to eight months.

Properties and medicinal uses: Spinach is highly nutritious and is particularly rich in antioxidants, especially when eaten fresh, steamed or lightly boiled. It is a rich source of vitamins A, C, E, K, magnesium, manganese, betaine, iron, vitamin B2, calcium, potassium, vitamin B6, folic acid, copper, protein, phosphorus, zinc, niacin, selenium and omega-3 fatty acids.

Spinach is a rich source of beta carotene, lutein and xanthene, preventing vitamin A deficiency disease, itching eyes, eye ulcers and dry eyes.

Spinach has high content of potassium and low content of sodium and is beneficial to those suffering from high blood pressure. The folic acid in spinach helps reduce hypertension and relaxes the blood vessels, maintaining proper blood flow.

Another component of spinach, C0-Q10, is an antioxidant and plays a vital role in strengthening the muscles, especially the heart muscle, which continuously pumps blood to all parts of the body.

Planting time and harvesting: Spinach is best grown in soil that is slightly heavy, as dry light soils can make the spinach run prematurely to seed, especially in hot weather. Sow the seeds in well-prepared and manured soil in 2.5 cm deep drills, with rows 30 cm apart. Thin the plants to 15 cm apart as soon as they are big enough to be handled.

Sow round seeded spinach every two weeks from mid-March to mid-July, with a sowing in mid-August of the winter prickly seeded type. Keep the plants well-watered in dry weather.

Part used: Green leaves

Preparation: Allow 2lbs of fresh spinach for four portions. Use well-developed, crisp, green young leaves. Wash the spinach at least twice, using salty water for the first wash. Remove any coarse main ribs from the leaves. Cook lightly in water or steam the leaves and add to salad or meat dishes. Do not overcook spinach.

Spring onions (scallions) – *Allium fistulosum*

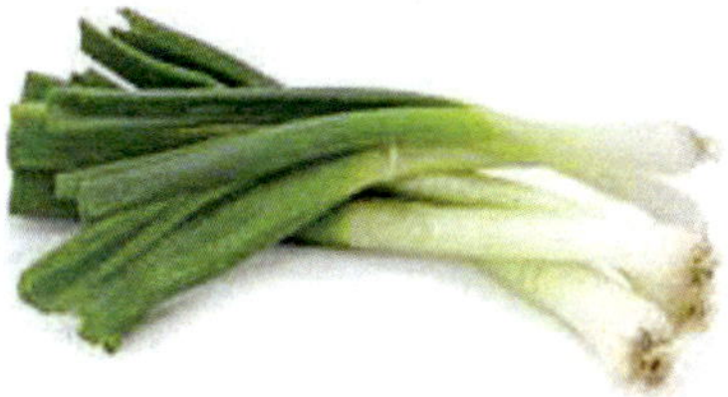

Spring onions (also known as scallions) are the edible plants of the *Allium* species. 'Scallion' is also a term used for young plants of the common onion (*A. cepa*) and shallot (*A. cepa* var. *aggregatum*), which are harvested before the bulbs form or when slight bulbing has occurred. Grown for their taste, they are milder than most onions.

Properties and medicinal uses: Spring onions reduce cholesterol levels and lower blood pressure, therefore reducing the risk of coronary heart disease. They also contain substances that prevent the formation of blood clots (in smaller amounts than regular onions, but still useful).

Planting time and harvesting: Sow main crop onion seeds from late February to early April for an August or September crop. Sow the seeds very thinly into drills 13 mm deep, in rows 23 cm apart. Carefully cover the seeds with soil and gently water in. Germination will take place after approximately 21 days.

Thin out the seedlings to 2.5 cm-5 cm apart when they have pushed through the soil and are standing vertically, and then again later to 10 cm apart.

Transplant them 10 cm apart, in rows 23 cm apart. Transplant the seedlings firmly, ensuring the roots fall into the bottom of the hole and are not gathered up around the onion bulb area. The base of the onions should be 13 mm deep.

Part used: Bulb, green leaves.

Preparation: Cut at root level. Wash them well, trim off the root and tops and remove any loose layers of skin. Spring onions can be eaten cooked or raw in salads. Diced spring onions can be used in soup, noodles, sandwiches, curries and stir-fries.

Sunflower – *Helianthus annuus*

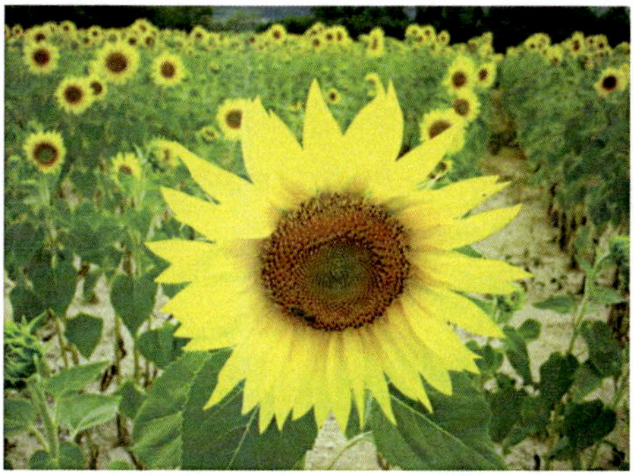

The sunflower is an annual plant native to the Americas. It can grow to heights of 1.5-3.5 metres and has a rough, hairy stem, coarsely toothed leaves and a circular head of flowers. The head consists of 1-2,000 individual flowers joined together by a receptacle base.

Properties and medicinal uses: Sunflower seeds are rich in a number of nutrients that protect against cardiovascular and other diseases and act as antioxidants and anti-carcinogens, including vitamin E, betaine, phenolic acids, choline, arginine and lignans.

Sunflower oil is used in massage treatments on mature skin to relax and hydrate the skin.

Planting time and harvesting: Sunflowers need full sun and grow best in fertile, moist, well-drained soil with plenty of mulch. Make sure the spot you choose is sheltered from strong winds and is close to a fence so the stems can be tied securely.

Soak your seeds the night before planting in a little warm water. Dig some holes and plant the seeds around 5 cm deep and 15 cm apart.

About 2 weeks later you should see some shoots coming through. If they are being attacked by garden pests, cover them with a plastic cup with the bottom cut off. If the sunflowers begin to bend over as they grow, tie them up.

To harvest, wait until the sunflower heads have gone completely brown on the plant, then chop them off with enough stem to hang them up to dry out for 2 weeks. Once dry, rub the heads together to loosen the seeds. Put around 50 or so seeds aside in a marked envelope to use the following year.

Part used: Seeds, oil.

Preparation: Sunflower seeds add crunch, taste and nutrition to a variety of foods. Toss them over salad, mix them in breakfast cereals and smoothies or add them to your home-baked, whole grain breads. Sunflower seeds are also sold as a pre-roasted snack food.

Sunflower oil, extracted from the seeds, is used for cooking and to produce margarine as it is cheaper than olive oil.

Tomato – *Solanum lycopersicum*

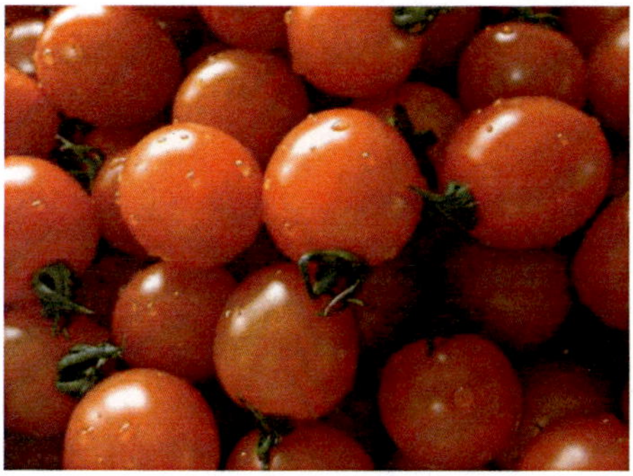

The tomato is a savoury fruit belonging to the *Nightshade* family, and is native to South America. Its many varieties are now grown around the world, often in greenhouses in cooler climates. The plant typically grows to 1-3 metres in height and has a weak stem that requires support.

Properties and medicinal uses: The consumption of the tomato is believed to benefit the heart and other organs. Tomatoes contain vitamins A, B, C, K, lycopene, thiamin, calcium, iron, phosphorus, potassium and protein. Lycopene, one of the most powerful natural antioxidants, has been shown to enhance the skin's ability to protect against harmful UV rays. Tomato consumption has been associated with decreased risk of breast cancer, head and neck cancers and might be strongly protective against neurodegenerative diseases. It is also a good blood purifier and helps in cases of congestion of the liver as well as for dissolving gallstones. The tomato is a natural antiseptic and can help protect against infection. The nicotinic acid in tomatoes reduces blood cholesterol and the vitamin K helps prevent haemorrhages.

Planting time and harvesting: Tomato plants will flourish indoors on a sunny windowsill or in a greenhouse (and can even be transplanted outside in the warmest months). Fill a 7.5 cm pot with compost, lightly firm and water. Then scatter 4-5 seeds evenly on the soil and cover with a further thin layer of soil. Place on a windowsill to germinate (which will take about 2 weeks).

After about 8 weeks, the seedlings should be large enough to be moved into their separate pots. Hold a seedling gently by its leaves and carefully lever up. Take another 7.5 cm pot filled with compost, make a hole in the centre of the soil and carefully lower in the seedling. Gently firm down, making sure the roots are covered and water. When the roots come through the drainage hole, repeat the process and transplant each seedling into a 12.5 cm pot. As the plants grow, snap out any shoots that appear in the leaf joints. When each plant has produced 4 sets of flowering trusses, pinch out the growing tip. Water the plants daily and once flowers have started to appear, feed with a tomato fertiliser every week.

Part used: Fruit.

Preparation: The tomato can be used in various ways, including raw in salads, processed into ketchup, tomato soup and pickle, or juiced for a delicious drink (with a dash of Worcester sauce).

HERBS AND SPICES

Angelica – *Angelica archangelica*

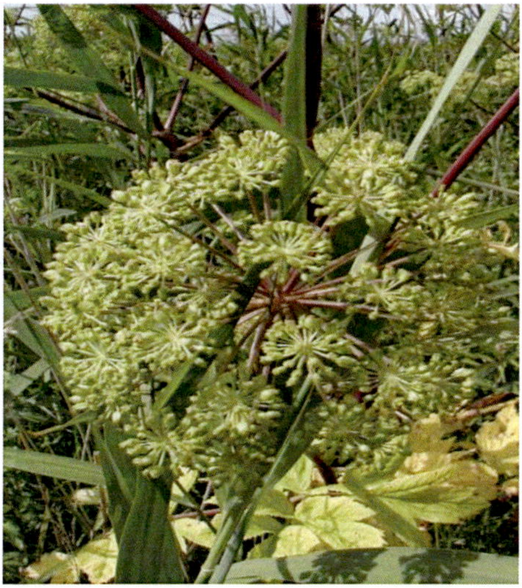

Angelica is a biennial plant from the *Apiaceae* family and is native to temperate and sub-arctic parts of the Northern Hemisphere where it grows wild. The roots of the angelica are poisonous but thoroughly drying them will eliminate the hazard. In the wild this herb resembles water hemlock, an extremely toxic plant. The two plants are very easy to confuse.

Properties and medicinal uses: Angelica is a good source of vitamins A, B1, B2, B3, folic acid, B12, E, iron, magnesium, potassium and zinc.

Research has shown that angelica has anti-inflammatory effects, which can be used in the treatment of arthritis, as well as increasing red blood cell counts, which could be beneficial in treating anaemia. It is also believed to increase the ability to clot blood; however, *anyone at risk of heart disease should avoid this herb.* Further research indicates that angelica relaxes the intestines, thus easing colic and flatulence. It also acts as a urinary antiseptic in cases of cystitis.

Angelica is an effective expectorant for asthma, bronchitis, coughs and pleurisy, particularly when accompanied by colds, flu or a high temperature.

Drinking angelica tea will result in local anaesthesia. Externally, angelica can be used as a poultice for eyes and as a hot compress for gout.

Planting time and harvesting: Angelica thrives in a moist, rich, slightly acid soil, and a semi-shaded location. Sow the seeds within a few weeks of ripening or they will not germinate.

Sow the seeds in autumn or spring, 13 mm deep in well-prepared beds, allowing 60 cm in each direction. Cover the seeds with a thin layer of fine soil. Germination should take about a month.

Angelica is a biennial herb; however, it will continue to live for several more years if you nip off the flower stems before they bloom. Harvest the stalks in the second season and the seeds as soon as they are ripe.

Part used: Roots, leaves, seeds.

Preparation: The roots, leaves and stalks of angelica can be used in various ways. The stems can be candied and used to decorate cakes and pastries. The boiled roots and stems can be eaten like celery. The seeds and oil made from the stems and roots are used as flavouring in many liqueurs such as vermouth, chartreuse, and Benedictine. The seeds also can be brewed into a healthy tea.

Borage – *Borago officinalis*

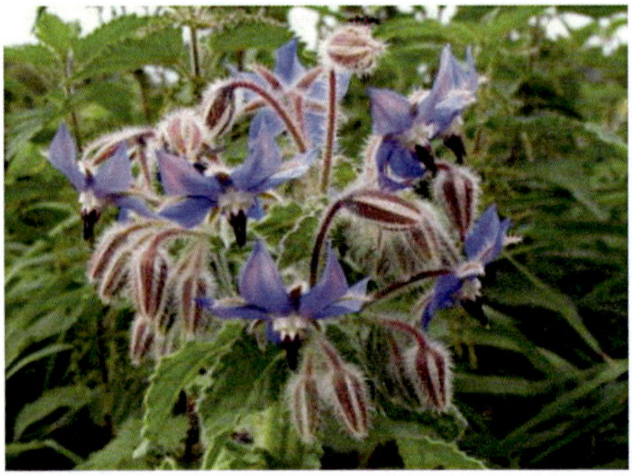

Copyright © 2010 Anemone Projectors

Borage, also known as starflower, is an annual herb native to Syria. In milder climates borage will bloom continuously for most of the year. Its oil is used to make 'Starflower Oil' capsules, which are sold in many shops as a herbal remedy to ease PMS, decrease inflammation and lower blood pressure.

Properties and medicinal uses: Borage contains vitamins A, B1, B2, B3, B6, B9 and C, as well as protein, calcium, iron, magnesium, manganese, phosphorus, potassium, sodium, zinc, copper, selenium, natural fats, and omega 6 fatty acids. These nutrients help to improve eyesight, fight viral infections, moisturize the mucous membranes, improve wound healing, prevent cell damage, improve dental health, improve the immune system, lower risks of some cancers, improve absorption of iron, improve lung health, prevent frequent colds, prevent frequent infections, improve oxygen distribution, provide energy, reduce fatigue and weakness, improve concentration, lower chances of headaches, lower risks of depression, support strong bones, regulate blood sugar levels, support healthy thyroid glands, improve nerve health, regulate cholesterol levels, and ease dizziness.

Planting time and harvesting: Borage is very easy to grow. It thrives in herb gardens or containers, but has a tendency to spread rapidly. Choose a sunny, sheltered location with well-manured and well-drained soil. When all frosts have ended, rake over the site to ensure it is level and scatter seeds over the surface. Rake the soil back over the seeds and water well. As it grows, thin out the seedlings to 30 cm apart and water in dry weather.

To prevent borage from self-seeding all over your garden, harvest the seeds to sow the following year. When the flowers have turned brown the seeds are ready; simply pick them off the plant and leave in a dry place such as a brown paper bag. They can be scattered over a prepared site the following spring.

Part used: Leaves, seeds, oil.

Preparation: Borage is often eaten as a fresh vegetable in soups, salads, sauces and pasta. Borage flower tastes like honey and is often used for decorating desserts.

To make borage tea, boil 2½ cups of water. Remove from the heat and add ¼ cup of dried leaves. Cover and allow the infusion to steep for 10 minutes. Drink ¼ cup of borage tea 3 times daily.

Chives – *Allium schoenoprasum*

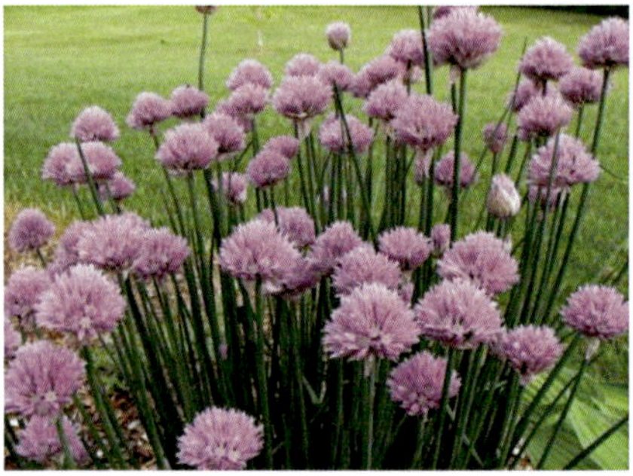

Copyright © 2009 Captain-tucker

The chive is the smallest member of the *Allium* family and is native to Europe, Asia and North America. It is grown for its leaves, which are used in cooking to add a very mild, onion-like flavour. The chive also acts as an insect repellent, making it useful in the common garden.

Properties and medicinal uses: The medicinal values of chives are similar to those of garlic but to a lesser degree. Chives are rich in vitamins A and C, contain trace amounts of sulphur, and are rich in calcium and iron. They are believed to have a beneficial effect on the circulatory system.

Planting time and harvesting: Sow the seeds in pots at a depth of 13 mm and water in. Place the pots in a moist, dark warm place to ensure germination (with chives this can be a slow process).

When the seedlings are 4 weeks old, transplant them in groups into shallow drills in a sunny part of the garden.

When the tops wither, divide the chive clumps into 5 cm segments (if they get too large, the centres may die out). Add decayed manure to the soil occasionally and keep well-watered for fuller plants.

To harvest, the leaves can be snipped when plants are around 15 cm in height. Do not cut closer than 5 cm from the ground, as the plants need some leaves to keep growing.

Part used: Leaves, flowers.

Preparation: Wash well. Chives are typically finely chopped and added to salads, omelettes, soups, chicken and fish.

Coriander – *Coriandrum sativum*

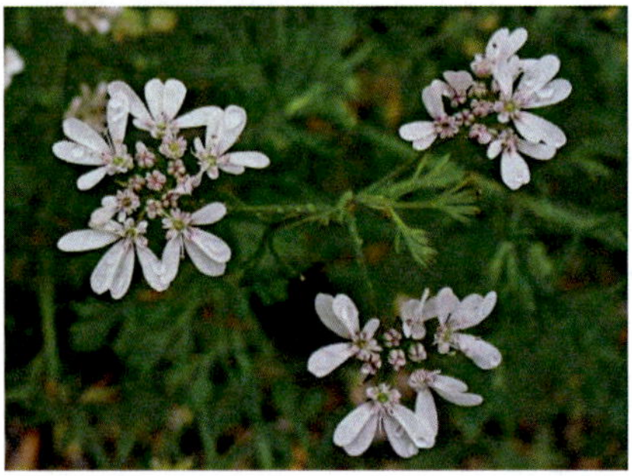

Copyright © 2009 H Zell

Coriander is a member of the *Apiaceae* family and native to southern Europe and North Africa to southwestern Asia. When fresh, its fruit is pungent but, once dried, it leaves a sweet and spicy aroma. Coriander is both a herb and a spice since both its leaves and its seeds are used as a seasoning condiment.

Properties and medicinal uses: Coriander is an excellent source of magnesium and manganese. Both its leaves and seeds contain antioxidants but the leaves have a more potent effect. The leaves have also been shown to have antibacterial activity against Salmonella.

Research has indicated that coriander lowers cholesterol levels, and also that it has both insulin-releasing and insulin-like activity. However, coriander is not suitable for everyone as it capable of producing an allergic reaction.

Planting time and harvesting: Coriander does not like being transplanted, so it is best to sow the seeds directly in the garden, in well-drained, weed-free, aerated soil, in a warm and light location.

Sow in May to ensure when soil temperatures are warm, which will promote more successful germination. Sow the seeds in drills around 1 cm deep and 4 cm apart, in rows 35 cm apart. Cover with soil and water in. Once the seedlings are about 4-5 cm in height, thin them down to 20 cm apart. Sow coriander seeds every few weeks to ensure a continuous crop through the season.

To harvest, pick mature leaves as and when required. Regular harvesting will postpone flowering. Once the plants do flower, allow them to set seed. The seed is ripe when it stops smelling unpleasant. Collect and use as required, keeping some to sow for another crop.

Part used: Fresh leaves, dried seeds.

Preparation: Wash well. Chopped coriander leaves can be used to garnish dishes such as dhal and curries. Add to the dish immediately before serving. Coriander leaves are often used in salads.

Curry leaf – *Murraya koenigii*

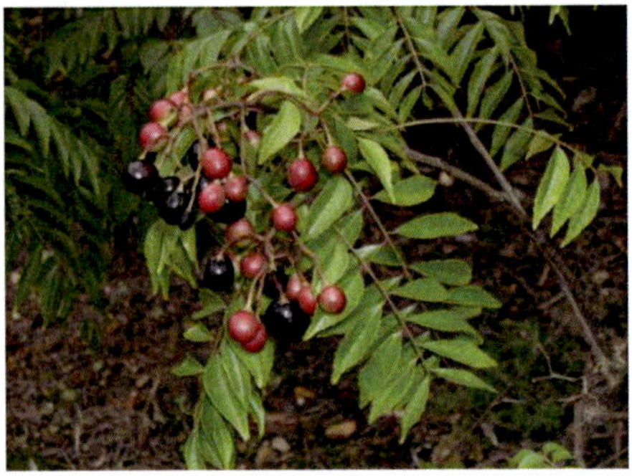

The curry leaf is an aromatic deciduous shrub and native to India, Sri Lanka, Bangladesh and the Andaman Islands.

Properties and medicinal uses: Special compounds in the curry leaf have been found that might make it an effective new medicine for diabetes sufferers.

Once consumed, the leaves stimulate the digestive system, and improve the quality of digestive enzymes and fluids that break down food. A small glass of buttermilk, seasoned with freshly chopped curry leaves, is a natural cure for nausea and/or vomiting. Curry leaves can also help get rid of indigestion and heartburn by adding a few drops of Manuka honey or lime juice, plus ½ teaspoon of crushed curry leaves, to a small glass of water.

Just 8-10 curry leaves in the daily diet can also help those wishing to lose weight. Properties in the leaves are known to flush out fat and toxins, thus reducing not only fat deposits laid up in the body but high cholesterol levels. Chop the leaves finely, mix into a drink or sprinkle over food.

Planting time and harvesting: Sow the seeds indoors during February/March. Fill a seed tray with compost and sow one seed in each cell at a depth of 13 mm. Moisten the soil with a light mist of water and place the tray in a warm location (approximately 20°C) in bright, indirect sunlight. Keep the soil moist while the seeds are germinating, which should take 2-3 weeks. Maintain temperature and exposure to sunlight as the seedlings grow.

Transplant the seedlings outdoors after the last frost. Dig the holes for the seedlings slightly wider than their root balls. Space the holes 30 cm apart. Remove the curry leaf plants from their containers and set one plant in each hole. Backfill each hole, pat the soil gently around each plant to remove air pockets and water generously. Give the plants at least 2.5 cm of water a week in lieu of rain, keeping the soil moist to a 2.5 cm depth at all times as the plants grow.

Spreading a 7.5 cm layer of straw or pine bark around the plants will improve drainage, reduce the chance of weeds and protect the roots of the plants during extreme temperature changes.

Part used: Leaves.

Preparation: Wash thoroughly. The leaves provide flavouring for curries, vegetable, fish and meat dishes, soups, chutneys, scrambled eggs and curry powder blends.

Dill – *Anethum graveolens*

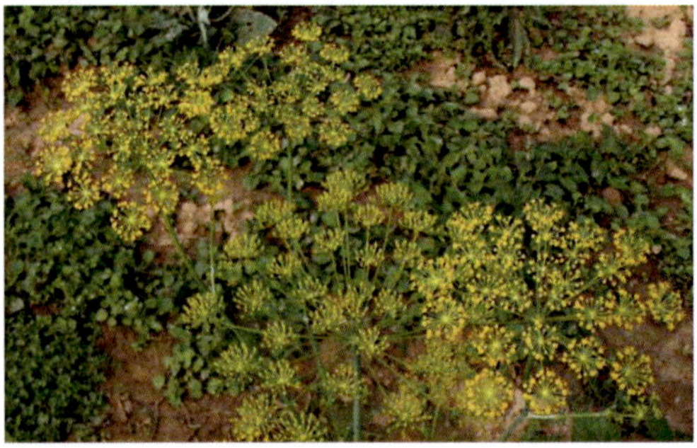

Copyright © 2005 Markus Hagen locher

Dill is a perennial herb, native to southwest Asia and now widely cultivated around the world. It has delicate, feathery leaves, topped with tiny clusters of yellow flowers.

Properties and medicinal uses: Dill is an excellent source of minerals, vitamins A, B and C, flavonoids, iron, dietary fibre, calcium, phosphor and magnesium. It has many medicinal properties and has been used as a health cure for thousands of years.

Dill is a relaxant, helping to ensure a good night's sleep. It strengthens the body, has diuretic properties that flush out toxins, aids digestion, eases painful wind and diarrhoea and calms the stomach, prevents cramp, ensures good bone and dental health, and freshens the breath.

The flavonoids in dill can help maintain regular menstrual cycles and also clear congestion in the respiratory system due to allergies or coughs. Its anti-oxidant properties fight free radicals and help protect against cancer.

Planting time and harvesting: Dill thrives in full sunshine, rich, well-drained soil and shelter from the wind. (Do not plant in partial shade as this could severely affect the crop.) Dill has long roots that need plenty of room to grow, so dig the soil to approximately 1½ spades deep. In April (after the last frost) sprinkle the seeds thinly in drills about 30-38 cm apart, and cover lightly with soil. The seedlings will start to appear about 2 weeks later, at which time thin them out to 24 cm apart. Ensure the bed is kept free of weeds and watered in dry conditions. Additional sowings can be made throughout spring and early summer to extend harvest time.

Harvest the seeds by cutting off the flower heads when the seeds begin to ripen. Place the seed heads upside down in a paper bag and leave in a warm dry place for around 7 days, after which time the seeds will separate easily. Stored in an airtight container, the seeds are viable for 3-10 years.

The leaves can be harvested after 8 weeks' growth by cutting the plant down to within 2.5 cm of its base. Once the flower heads appear, leaf production will cease.

Part used: Leaves, stems, seeds, oil.

Preparation: Dill is an aromatic herb that can be used to flavour a variety of dishes, such as rice, white fish, potatoes, broad beans and creamy sauces etc. It is best used fresh, as it loses its flavour if dried.

Echinacea – *E. purpurea, E. angustifolia*

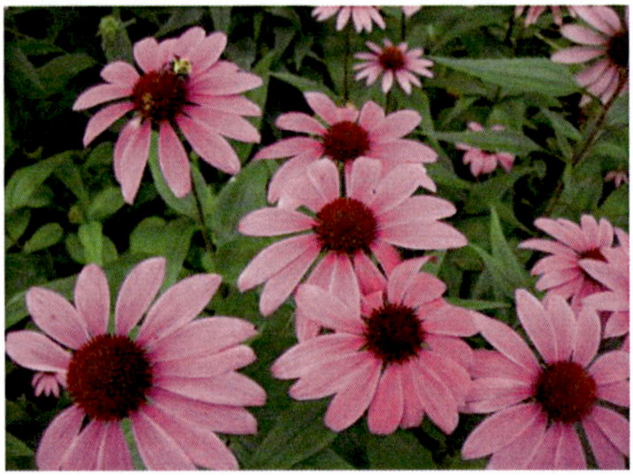

Echinacea is a herbaceous flowering plant of the *Asteraceae* family and native to north America. It is widely used in herbal medicine as well as being popular with gardeners for its beautiful flowers.

Properties and medicinal uses: The power of echinacea to cure the common cold is an ongoing subject of debate. Several trials showed that echinacea reduced the odds of developing a cold by 58% and the duration of a cold by 1-4 days. However, experts have disputed these findings.

Echinacea contains a variety of chemicals such as polysaccharides, glycoproteins, alkamides, volatile oils, and flavonoids, each of which plays a role in its curative effects. However, chemicals found in the root differ significantly from those in the upper part of the plant. For example, the roots have high levels of volatile oils while the visible parts of the plant contain more polysaccharides, which activate the immune system. These substances working together are what give echinacea its beneficial effects. Science has confirmed the roots as being anti-inflammatory, antibiotic, antiseptic, and a digestive treatment. The whole plant is considered beneficial in the external treatment of eczema, psoriasis, inflammatory skin conditions, sores, wounds, burns, and sore throat.

Planting time and harvesting: Echinacea will tolerate a wide variety of growing conditions but appreciates a partly shaded, warm spot in the garden. Sow the seeds in spring when the frosts have ended. Rake the surface of the soil and sprinkle the seeds; after they begin to germinate (10-20 days) lightly cover the seeds with about 4 mm of soil. When the seedlings are large enough to handle, thin them out to 55-60 cm apart and keep their plot weed free.

Allow echinacea plants to grow for 3-4 years before harvesting; meanwhile, they will bloom from June-October and will attract butterflies and be an asset to any garden.

The flowers should be harvested in full bloom in mid-July. The end of summer is the best time to harvest the seed heads for seed, when the stalks are brown and brittle. Harvest the echinacea roots in autumn, after the first frost. Dry the plant material fast and cool (artificially).

Part used: Root, rhizomes, above-ground parts.

Preparation: Traditionally used in decoctions, infusions, liquid extracts, powders, tablets and tinctures in herbal remedies.

Evening primrose - *Oenothera biennis*

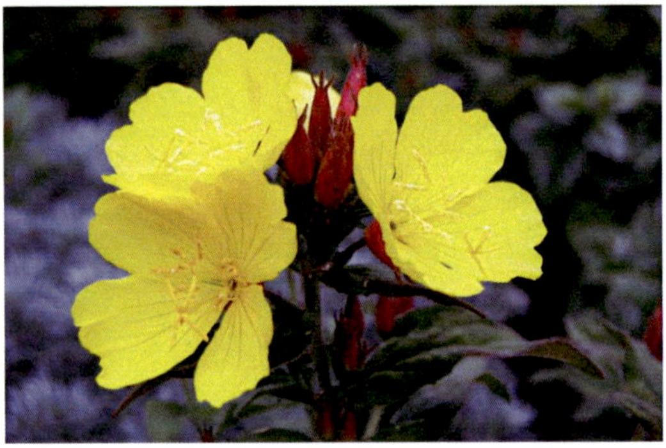

Copyright © 2009 UpstateNYer

Evening primrose *(Oenothera biennis)* is an annual/biennial flowering plant that is native to North America. It can grow to 30-150 cm tall and from late spring to late summer produces flowers that are pale yellow, 2.5-5 cm diameter, with four petals. The flowers open in the evening (hence its name 'Evening primrose') and close again around mid-morning the following day.

Properties and medicinal uses: Mature Evening primrose seeds contain approximately 7-10% gamma-linolenic acid, a rare essential fatty acid. Gamma-linolenic acid has shown potential in the fight against breast cancer and notably in pancreatic cancer.

The seed oil is used internally for alcohol-related liver damage, eczema, hyperactivity in children, multiple sclerosis, premenstrual and menopausal syndromes, and rheumatoid arthritis. Evening primrose oil can also be used externally for dry skin.

Planting time and harvesting: Evening primrose is a very easy plant to cultivate, and grows well in a sandy, light soil with full sunlight or light shade. At the beginning of spring (just before the last frost), spread the seeds approximately 10 cm apart and cover lightly with soil. As long as the area is not too wet, the seeds will happily grow. When the seedlings appear, provide a trellis or some form of support for it to cling to. Water during dry months and provide manure in spring. Prune the plants once flowering has completed and divide cuttings in the spring. Evening primrose will re-seed itself wherever it is planted.

Part used: Roots, shoots and seeds for oil.

Preparation: Young roots can be used as a vegetable and have a peppery flavour; shoots can be added to salads; and the seeds pressed to produce Evening primrose oil, a commonly used health supplement.

Hyssop – *Hyssopus officinalis*

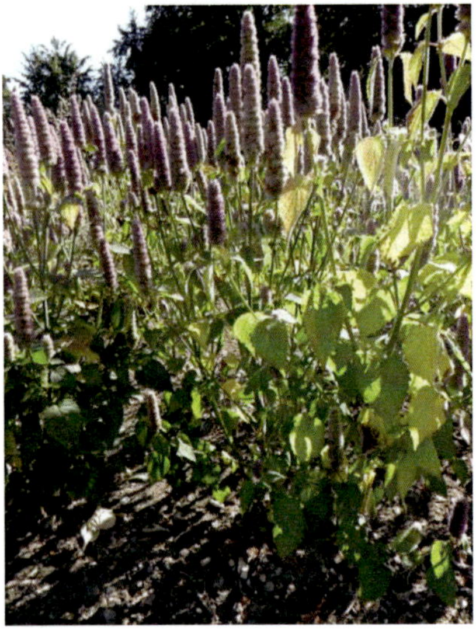

Copyright © 2009 Magnus Manske

Hyssop is an aromatic, herbaceous plant of the *Lamiaceae* family and is native to the Mediterranean and Asia. It has upright branched stems, narrow leaves, and develops small blue flowers during summer. It is widely cultivated as an ornamental plant, a herbal remedy and for culinary purposes.

Properties and medicinal uses: Hyssop is an excellent herb for easing respiratory ailments. It is also antibacterial, anti-inflammatory, anti-viral, and antiseptic and can help with innumerable medical conditions, including bronchitis, the common cold, insomnia, oedema, etc. When consumed as a tincture or tea, hyssop acts as an expectorant for the relief of congestion, aids digestion, regulates blood pressure, and eases painful wind. It also helps with circulatory problems, jaundice, liver and gallbladder complaints, gout and epilepsy. A poultice made up of ground leaves and used externally can help to heal wounds and bruises.

However, despite its many wonderful healing properties, hyssop should not be consumed by expectant mothers.

Planting time and harvesting: Hyssop should be grown in full sun on well-drained soil. Sow the seeds indoors in pots about 8-10 weeks before the last frost, planting the seeds just beneath the surface of the soil. Hyssop seeds usually take 14-21 days to germinate and can be transplanted in the garden in spring, after the last frost, spacing the seedlings about 15-30 cm apart. Hyssop does not require much watering but will benefit from occasional clipping.

To harvest, cut the plants on a dry day. Gather into small bunches and hang them upside down in a dark, well-ventilated place for about 5-6 days. When dried, store them in a dry, airtight container and they should keep for 12-18 months.

Part used: Leaves, flowers, oil.

Preparation: Hyssop leaves have a slightly bitter, minty taste and can be added to soups, salads or meats. But use them sparingly, as they are very strong. Hyssop oil is used in Aromatherapy treatment.

Lady's mantle – *Alchemilla vulgaris*

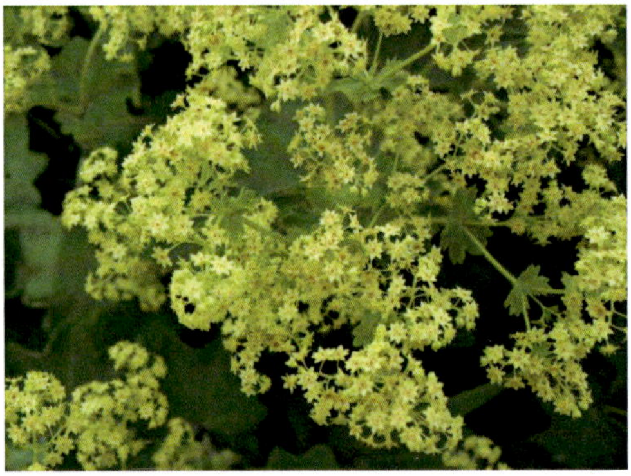

Copyright © 2008 Anneli Salo

Lady's mantle is a herbaceous perennial plant of the *Rosaceae* family and is native to Europe, Asia, and North America. It is often cultivated for its glorious foliage and flowers, as well as for culinary and medical purposes.

Properties and medicinal uses: When taken as an infusion of the dried herb, lady's mantle can help with lack of appetite, diarrhoea, enteritis, vomiting, rheumatism, and excessive menstrual bleeding. Its styptic properties help blood to clot and can be useful for internal bleeding or as a mouth wash after having teeth extracted. Used externally, this herb makes an excellent douche for leucorrhoea, and an ideal cleanser or poultice for wounds. There is also an old belief that if you put lady's mantle under your pillow before going to sleep, it will give you a restful night.

Planting time and harvesting: Lady's mantle is a hardy plant that grows best in moist conditions and fertile soil; however, it will tolerate most types of soil. A sunny location with partial shade will give optimum results. In March, plant the seeds indoors 4 mm deep, in pots filled with compost. Water in and keep in a warm environment (16-20°C) until germination in 3-4 weeks' time.

After the last frost and when the seedlings are large enough to handle, transplant them into the garden. Dig a trench, adding a little organic fertilizer; place each seedling 45 cm apart and no deeper than they were in their pots; add mulch around the seedlings with 7.5 cm of organic compost. Water well until the soil is completely moist. Note that the plants will not bloom for 2 years.

Apply organic fertilizer lightly to the top of the soil each year in early spring and mulch again as above. If plants become too crowded, thinning them out can also be done in spring. Do not over-water in warmer weather, as lady's mantle is quite tolerant of dry conditions.

Harvest the whole plant in June and July when in flower, and when the leaves are at their best, and dried.

Part used: Leaves, flower, rootstock.

Preparation: The root and leaves of lady's mantle are edible but high in tannins. This is okay, but not if eaten to excess.

Lavender – *Lavandula angustifolia*

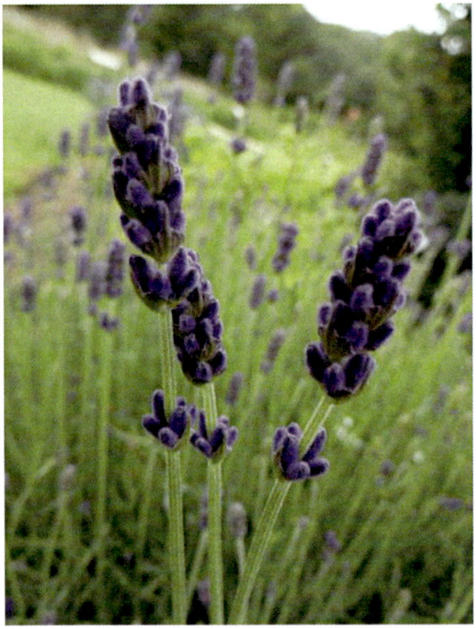

Copyright © 2010 Magnus Manske

English lavender is a member of the *Lamiaceae* family and is prized by gardeners for its fragrance and colour. Lavender essential oil is included in many preparations, such as balms, salves, perfumes, cosmetics, and topical applications. Its flowers are often used in sachets to freshen clothes and linen, and are also added to pot-pourri.

Properties and medicinal uses: Lavender oil has antiseptic and anti-inflammatory properties and is often used in aromatherapy. If diluted to 1 part lavender oil to 10 parts water, it can help clear acne and soothe insect bites and burns. A little oil applied to the temples can ease headaches and aid restful sleep.

Planting time and harvesting: Lavender is best grown from existing plants rather than seed. It flourishes in a sunny, partly shaded location with good air circulation, in well-drained, sandy or gravelly soil. Plant the lavender in April or May, 90 cm apart, making sure to loosen the roots before placing in the soil; water at the time of planting and each day until they are established. Lavenders should be pruned once a year, in late summer, to keep them in shape.

Harvest the lavender in late June/early July, in the early morning, when the dew is off them. Select stems that only have 1 or 2 opened flower buds, tie them together in bunches and hang upside down in a dry, airy space.

Part used: Flowers, leaves.

Preparation: Lavender flowers are a rich source of nectar from which bees make a high-quality honey. The flowers are sometimes used as cake decorations. Lavender is often used to flavour desserts and, with its floral, slightly sweet taste, goes well with chocolate. It is only from the buds that lavender oil can be extracted.

Lemon balm – *Melissa officinalis*

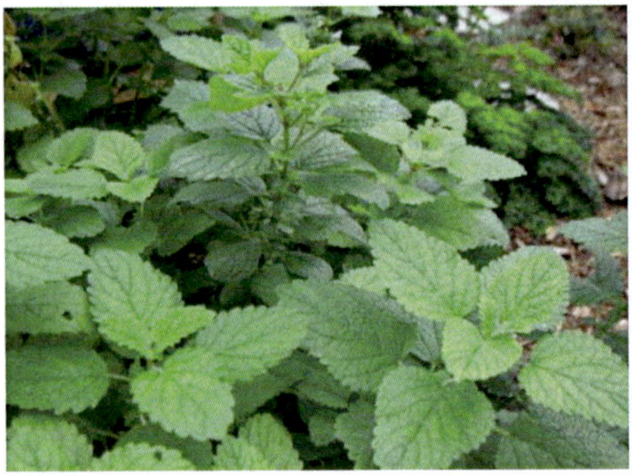

Copyright © 2009 Datkins

Lemon balm is a perennial herb from the mint family *Lamiaceae*, native to Europe, Asia, and Africa. Its leaves are lemon scented and its small white flowers attract bees and butterflies.

Properties and medicinal uses: Lemon balm is a source of flavonoids, polyphenols, tannins, volatile oil and triterpenes. It has antispasmodic, carminative and antiviral properties. Lemon balm can have a considerable effect on insomnia and anxiety, promoting calm and restful sleep. It has also been shown to be a mood enhancer and to increase alertness. Various studies have found that lemon balm can help sufferers of Alzheimer's disease by improving cognitive function and decreasing agitation. Lemon balm works well as a treatment for viral cold sores, and when rubbed on the skin, the crushed leaves of the lemon balm act as a repellent for mosquitoes. However, despite its many healing properties, lemon balm should not be used by anyone taking thyroid medication.

Planting time and harvesting: Lemon balm requires fertile, well-drained sandy soil and a winter mulch, or adequate protection from snow, to thrive. It grows best in full sun but will tolerate moderate shade. Plant lemon balm seeds indoors about 6-8 weeks before the last frost by filling a seed tray with equal parts of potting soil and vermiculite. Water well and allow the tray to drain completely. Then scatter the seeds over the surface and cover lightly with 4 mm of soil. Lightly spray the surface of the soil with water, but do not disturb the seeds. Place the tray in a bright area, out of direct sunlight. Keep the soil moist with a misting spray while the seeds germinate (about 3 weeks). Transplant the seedlings when they have gained their third set of leaves.

Mix a 7.5 cm layer of well-rotted manure into the soil to a depth of 20 cm. Make planting holes that are the same depth as the seeding tray, 30-45 cm apart. Place the roots into the planting holes and pack the soil around them. Water the area with a fine mist until the top 10 cm of soil is moist. Keep the soil moist until the seedlings are established and begin to grow. Harvest leaves as required throughout the season. For larger cuttings, leave 5-10 cm above the soil surface. Lemon balm can be harvested several times each season through to November. To dry, hang in bunches in a warm, well-ventilated shed. When dry, store in tightly closed containers.

Part used: Leaves, oil.

Preparation: Lemon balm can be used as flavouring in ice cream and herbal teas. It is also a good addition to a fruit salad or as a seasoning for fish.

Lemon verbena – *Aloysia citrodora*

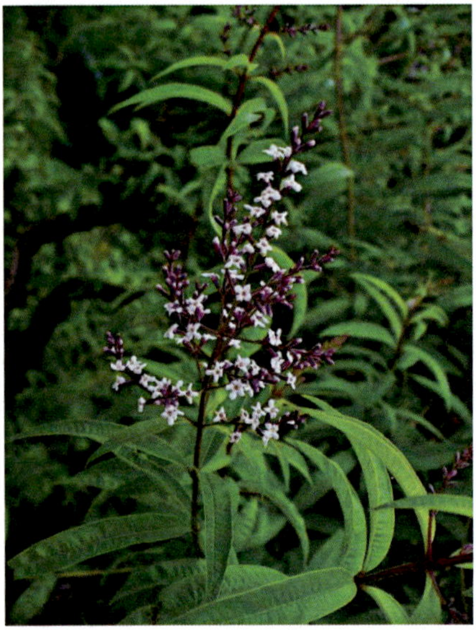

Lemon verbena is a deciduous perennial shrub from the *Verbenaceae* family and is native to South America. It has a lovely lemony scent, which becomes stronger when the leaves are crushed. Its oil has been used in cologne, toilet water, perfume, and soap. If grown below windows and near doorways, the plant will repel midges, flies and other insects.

Properties and medicinal uses: The chemical components of lemon verbena include borneol, geraniol, linalool, nerol, citral, dipentene, limonene and myrcene. It is an antiseptic, antispasmodic, digestive, emollient, febrifuge, hepatic, insecticide, sedative, stomachic and tonic. Lemon verbena's therapeutic properties are used to relieve stomach cramps, reduce fever, strengthen the nervous system and relieve stress. Used as a compress, its leaves can help reduce puffy eyes.

Steep lemon verbena leaves in hot water to make a relaxing and soothing tea to ease congestion and indigestion. The stimulant action on the digestive system helps to digest fats and is excellent for liver health. However, lemon verbena can irritate the stomach if taken long term.

Planting time and harvesting: Lemon verbena prefers a hot climate, so it is best grown from cuttings or seedlings obtained from a garden centre and grown indoors. When taking a cutting, choose a small sprig that includes a few leaves. Allow it to stand in a small glass of water until it sprouts roots at least 2.5 cm long then transfer it to a large pot containing good potting soil. As the plant grows, it may need to be re-potted into larger pots. This is the time to trim the roots to contain its growth.

When the plant reaches 15 cm or more in height, cut back the top by about 5 cm to encourage more side branches. Lemon verbena needs lots of water, so water at least twice a week. Do not let the soil dry out. Feed the plant with standard fertilizer twice a year, in spring and autumn, for optimal growth. Lemon verbena may lose its leaves in the winter; however, this does not mean that there is anything wrong with it. Water it once a week and it should revive in spring.

Harvest when required, leaving at least 2/3 of the leaves still on the plant to help it recover. Pick only the leaves and tender stem tips (older branches will not yield the characteristic lemon flavour). Lemon verbena will not lose its taste or fragrance if dried, and can be stored for many months.

Part used: Leaves, oil.

Preparation: Lemon verbena leaves can be used to flavour fish and poultry, vegetable marinades, salad dressings, jams, fruit salads and beverages. It also is used to make herbal teas, or added to ordinary tea in place of a slice of lemon.

Marjoram – *Origanum majorana*

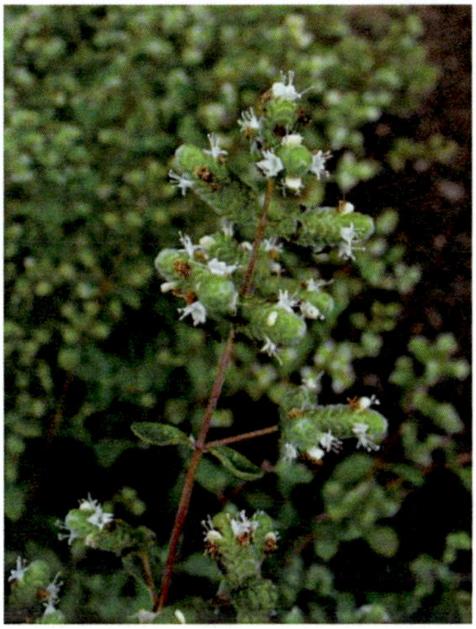

Copyright © 2009 H Zell

Marjoram is a member of the *Lamiaceae* family and is native to the Mediterranean. It is a perennial herb with sweet pine and citrus flavours.

Properties and medicinal uses: Marjoram has many chemical components, including borneol, camphor and pinene. The leaf of the marjoram acts as a decongestant and is used in cases of bronchitis, sinusitis and sinus headaches. It can also be used to soothe the nerves and reduce tension and stress, while its flavonoids help to relieve insomnia, tension headaches and migraines, prevent cholesterol build-up and improve blood circulation. Marjoram promotes healthy digestion and can be used to treat loss of appetite, indigestion, nausea and flatulence.

Marjoram also has anti-inflammatory properties and can be used internally or externally. Used externally, it alleviates aches and pains, soothes muscular pain, bruises, arthritis, sprains and stiff joints. Used internally, it eases severe stomach cramps, spasms and painful menstruation. Marjoram stimulates perspiration, which can help to reduce fevers and relieve cold and flu symptoms.

Planting time and harvesting: Marjoram thrives best in full sun, in light well-drained soil. The seeds can be sown directly outside in April. Sow them 2 cm deep and 15 cm apart. Thin to 30 cm apart when the seedlings appear two weeks later. Marjoram is tolerant of most conditions and requires little or no feeding. Make sure they do not dry out during the first few months, after which they are much hardier and will tolerate drought.

The leaves of a one year old plant can be harvested from June to November, as required. Harvest the leaves on a dry day and place them in a dark, dry, warm place until completely dried. When stored in an airtight container; they will keep their flavour for around 3 months.

Part used: Leaves, oil.

Preparation: Marjoram can be used as stuffing for chicken and turkey, and to enhance the flavour of carrot and squash when cooked with it. Its leaves can be used to make an excellent herbal tea with a variety of healing properties.

Marshmallow – *Althaea officinalis*

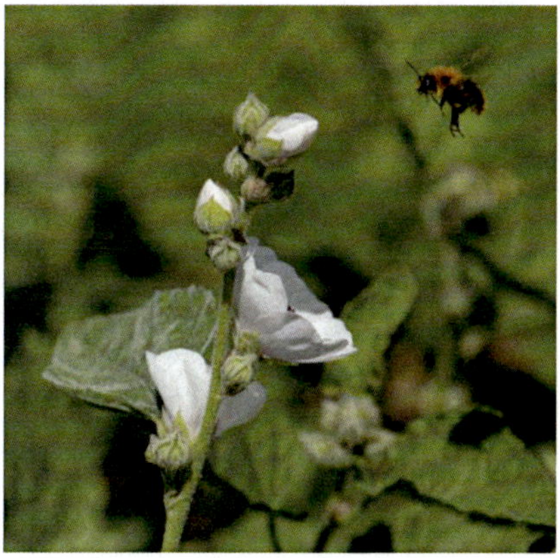

Copyright © 2007 Andre Karwath

Marshmallow is a hardy perennial and native to Africa. The name *Althaea* comes from the Greek word *altho,* meaning 'to cure'. It has been used since the time of the ancient Egyptians to make the sweets known today as 'marshmallow'.

Properties and medicinal uses: The leaves, flowers and root all have therapeutic properties. The leaves are used in ailments of the lungs and the urinary system, in particular urethritis and kidney stones. The root can be used to treat inflammation of the mouth, gastritis, peptic ulcers, enteritis and colitis. It can also increase the flow of breast milk, soothe the bronchial tubes, relieve constipation and treat irritable bowel syndrome. The root can also be used externally to treat varicose veins, ulcers, abscesses and boils. The flowers of the marshmallow root are used in the making of expectorant syrups. They are harvested when the plant is at least two years old, and in August just as the flower is coming into bloom. The flowers are also used as a cosmetic treatment for the skin.

Planting time and harvesting: Marshmallow prefers full sunlight and sandy soil. The seeds should be sown indoors before the last frost. First, stratify the seeds by placing a small amount of damp sand in a plastic bag and mixing the seeds with the sand. Allow them to stand at room temperature for a day to absorb the moisture then refrigerate for 4-6 weeks. Shake the bag occasionally and if you see germination taking place, plant them immediately.

Use a pot with good drainage; fill with potting soil and place the stratified seeds, plus the sand, on the top of the soil. Cover the seeds very lightly with compost and water in. Cover pots to keep in the moisture. Keep the container moist at all times and place in a sunny, cool spot. Transplant the seedlings after the last frost. Dig deeply and space them 15 cm apart. Keep them well-watered until they are adequately established. Thin the plants to 30 cm apart during the first year then 60 cm apart during the second year. Harvest the leaves as they are needed and before the plant blooms. After the flowers bloom they can be harvested for use.

Part used: Leaves, flowers, root.

Preparation: Marshmallow seeds can be eaten as a snack or sprinkled on salads like nuts. The flower is also edible and makes an interesting addition to any food dish. The leaves can be added to lettuce, or steamed and served as a vegetable. To eat the root, boil it to soften, then fry and add salt.

Meadowsweet – *Filipendula ulmaria*

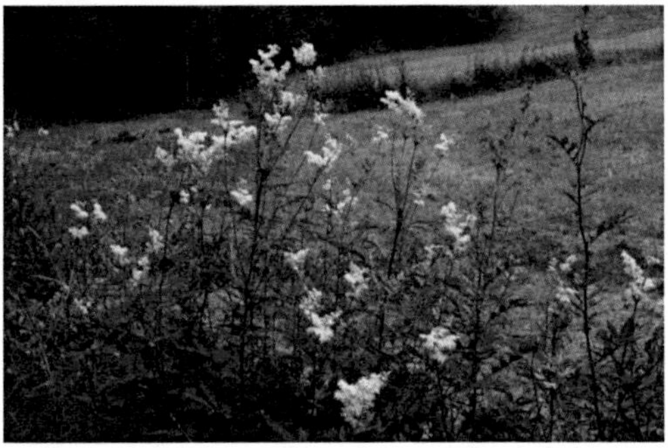

Copyright © 2009 Stobilomyces

Meadowsweet is a perennial herb and a member of the *Rosaceae* family. It is native to Europe and Western Asia. Meadowsweet has clusters of delicate, creamy-white flowers with a very strong, sweet smell.

Properties and medicinal uses: Meadowsweet's active ingredients include essential oils, flavonoids, phenolic glycosides, salicylic acid, and tannins. It is an anti-inflammatory, antiseptic, diaphoretic diuretic, haemostatic, sanative, stomachic, and tonic. The plant is traditionally used as a remedy for acidic stomach, diarrhoea, gastritis, heartburn, hyperacidity, and peptic ulcers, while its chemicals are used in the making of aspirin – chewing the peeled root is an old remedy for the relief of headaches. Meadowsweet is also a natural treatment for afflictions of the blood. It is also believed to be very effective against the pathogens that cause diphtheria, both amoebic and bacillary dysenteries, and pneumonia. The flowers, when made into tea, can help ease flu symptoms. However, anyone sensitive to aspirin should avoid meadowsweet.

Planting time and harvesting: Meadowsweet grows well in either full sun or partial shade, in moist and alkaline soil (try a spot near a pond or at the bottom of a slope). In autumn, sprinkle the seeds onto moist humus-rich potting compost in a seed tray and cover with a fine layer of compost. Place the tray under a cold frame to germinate in a temperature of 10-13°C. When seedlings emerge, transfer to separate pots using fresh potting compost with the same mix as before. Put the pots back under the cold frame during winter and keep the soil moist. In late spring, dig the soil over and add rich humus. Plant the seedlings in holes 30 cm apart, fill in and press gently around the plants to bed them in. Water at soil level to keep the ground moist. Cut off the flower spike before flowers appear in June if you want to keep the foliage full and bushy. Let the plant flower if you want seeds for growing new plants. Harvest seeds from the seed heads between August and September or let the plant seed itself naturally.

Part used: Dried flowers, leaves, root.

Preparation: The whole plant can be used to flavour wine, beer and many types of vinegar. The flowers can be added to stewed fruit and jams, giving them a mild almond flavour, and the leaves can be added to soups to intensify their flavour. Dried, the flowers make lovely pot-pourri.

Meadowsweet flowers can be made into a sachet or herb pillow and placed in drawers or cupboards to leave your clothes smelling fresh.

Mint – *Mentha spp*

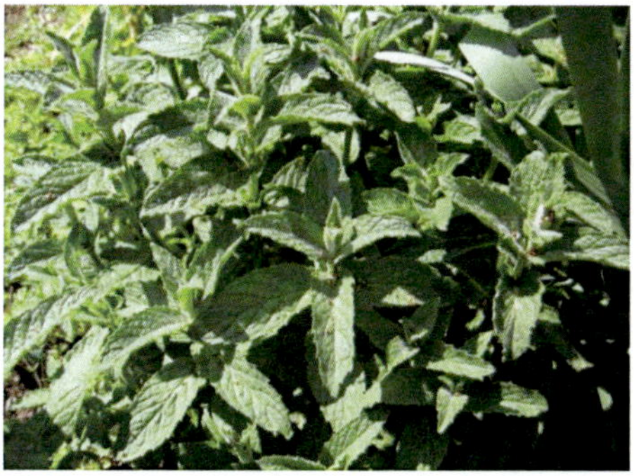

Copyright © 2005 Gogo

Mint is an aromatic member of the *Lamiaceae* family and native to Asia and the Mediterranean. Its flowers are white to purple and the fruit is a small, dry capsule containing 1-4 seeds.

Properties and medicinal uses: Mint contains manganese, iron, copper, potassium and calcium and is rich in vitamins A and C and has small amounts of vitamin B2. Vitamin C is an antioxidant, which may help to decrease the risk of colon and rectal cancer.

Mint can relieve symptoms of indigestion, heartburn and irritable bowel syndrome, inhibit the growth of many different types of bacteria and fungus, ease breathing and respiratory passages, relieve the symptoms of colds and flu, act as a mild sedative, relieve minor aches and pains, cure bad breath, treat minor burns and itching, and cleanse the blood. Mint tea can help clear up skin disorders such as acne.

Planting time and harvesting: Mint is best cultivated from the runners or roots of existing healthy plants and is easy to maintain.

It prefers a shady, moist location but will grow in partial sun. Pot a piece of root in a small container and keep it well-watered. Leaves should begin to sprout within a few weeks and can be transplanted into the garden the following spring. It is advisable to grow mint in a container to prevent its roots from spreading and damaging other plants. Do this by sinking the container into the soil so it appears that the plant is part of the herb bed; the roots will be contained so the plant can never grow beyond the confines of the pot. Each plant should be placed at least 30 cm apart. Mint requires only occasional weeding and watering.

Mint can be harvested throughout summer as soon as the leaves are large enough to pick. Fresh mint leaves should be used immediately or stored up to a couple of days in plastic bags in the fridge. Dried mint leaves should be stored in an airtight container and placed in a cool, dark, dry area.

Part used: Leaves, oil.

Preparation: Mint leaves can be used in teas, beverages, jellies, syrups, sweets and ice creams. It can be used in a variety of dishes including roast lamb and salad and goes well with fresh peas.

Make tea from fresh or dried leaves for a tasty and refreshing after-dinner stomach soother.

Parsley – *Petroselinum crispum*

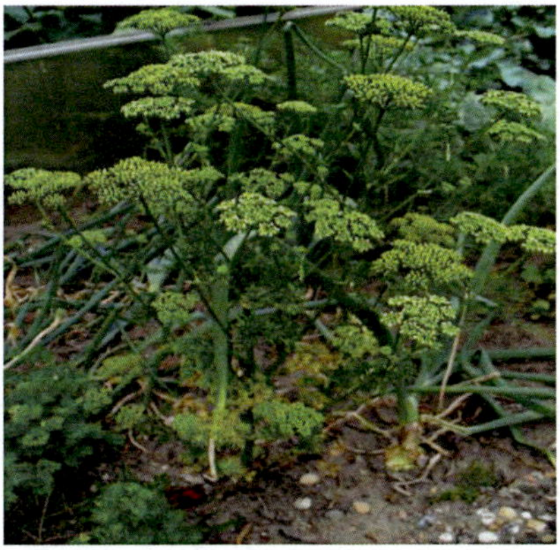

Copyright © 2009 H Zell

Parsley is a member of the *Apiacea* family and is native to the central Mediterranean region. It is a biennial herbaceous plant in milder climates and is widely cultivated as a herb, spice and vegetable.

Properties and medicinal uses: Parsley is a rich source of nutrients, including calcium, iron, and vitamins A, B, C, and K. Parsley enhances the body's ability to absorb manganese, which is important to help build strong bones. This is especially so when parsley is eaten together with foods rich in copper and zinc, e.g. shellfish and whole grains. Parsley tea can help control high blood pressure and also has diuretic properties. Parsley is believed to reduce itching of mosquito bites when crushed and rubbed on the skin, and freshen the breath when chewed.

Pregnant women should avoid eating parsley in excess as it can have uteronic effects. However, parsley is safe if eaten in normal quantities.

Planting time and harvesting: Parsley prefers a rich, well-dug soil that does not dry out too often, and a sunny location. It is often very slow to germinate, taking four to six weeks, as it needs high temperatures (ideally 20-30°C). So it is recommended that the seeds are sown in pots and kept indoors in a warm room until the seedlings have sprouted.

In March, sow four or five seeds in each pot and from those that germinate, choose the strongest and thin them out to one seedling per pot. When the seedlings are approximately 8 cm in height, prepare the soil outside by digging it well and adding plenty of organic matter. Add some bonemeal to the top layer of soil.

To keep the plants healthy, give them some general fertiliser once a month. When sown in March, parsley can normally be harvested from July to July the following year. Because it is a biennial, it will then produce seeds, which effectively ends the plant's use as a herb.

Part used: Leaves.

Preparation: Wash the leaves well and chop them. Sprinkle raw over salad or add to an omelette mix, rice, mashed potato, soups, spaghetti bolognese, meatballs, beefburgers, fish and chicken.

Rosemary – *Rosmarinus officinalis*

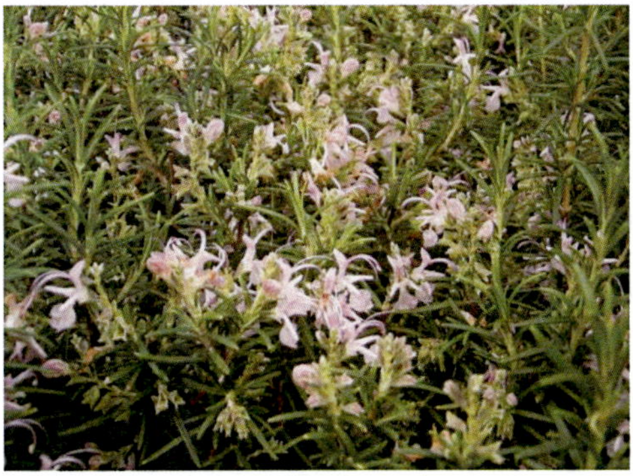

Copyright © 2008 Frank Vincentz

Rosemary is a woody, perennial member of the *Lamiaceae* family and is native to the Mediterranean region. Its flowers can be pink, white, purple or blue.

Properties and medicinal uses: Rosemary is high in iron, calcium and vitamin B6, and also contains carnosic acid and rosmarinic acid, camphor, caffeic acid, ursolic acid, betulinic acid, rosmaridiphenol, and rosmanol. Its carnosic acid is an antioxidant and may help lower the risk of strokes, Alzheimer's disease and Amyotrophic lateral sclerosis. Carnosol is also a promising cancer chemoprevention and anti-cancer agent, and is an anti-inflammatory

When rosemary is harvested properly and used within recommended guidelines, its side effects are minimal. However, rosemary should not be used by anyone suffering from epilepsy or anaemia.

Planting time and harvesting: Rosemary is harder to germinate than most herbs and is best propagated from cuttings. Take 8 cm cuttings from new growth in late spring (cutting just below a leaf joint). Put the cuttings in 7.5 cm pots filled with potting compost. Stand the pots in water to enable the compost to draw up the water. Once the compost is moist, place the pots under a windowsill propagator or clear plastic bottle to retain heat. The cuttings will be ready for transplanting about 2 months later.

Rosemary likes a lot of sunshine but will tolerate some shade and grows best in well-drained soil. When the seedlings are 7.5 cm in height, transplant into the garden by digging holes slightly larger than the size of the pots, spacing them about 60 cm apart. Add 1 cm of sandy soil or sharp sand to the bottom of the hole. Place the plants in the holes and fill around with a mix of half sharp sand and half from the removed soil. Put strong stakes in the ground and tie string round each stake and plant to support them in winter.

Harvest as and when required, being careful not to remove more than 20% of the growth at a time. To dry, cut branches before the plant flowers. Hang bundles upside down in an airy place and strip the leaves from the stem when dry.

Part used: Leaves, oil.

Preparation: Dried rosemary leaves can be added to soups, stews, meat, fish, salads, potato dishes, and used with garlic when roasting vegetables.

Sage – *Salvia officinalis*

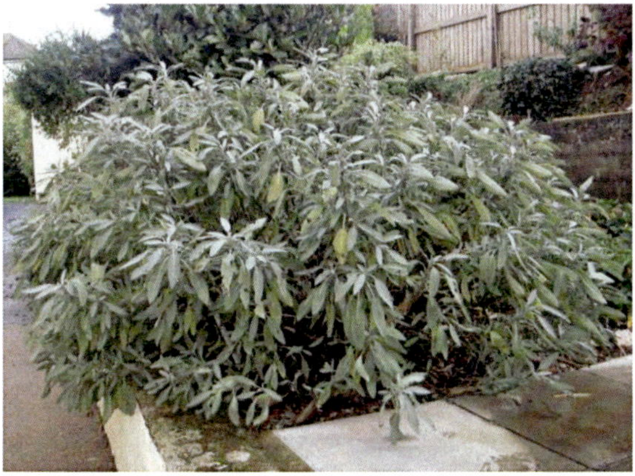

Copyright © 2006 Herbythyme

Sage is a perennial evergreen member of the *Lamiaceae* family and is native to the Mediterranean. Its flowers are usually lavender in colour but may be white, pink or purple.

Properties and medicinal uses: The most beneficial constituents of sage are found in its essential oil, which contains cineole, borneol, and thujone. Sage leaf also contains tannic acid, oleic acid, ursonic acid, ursolic acid, cornsole, cornosilic acid, fumaric acid, chlorogenic acid, caffeic acid, niacin, nicotinamide, flavones, flavonoid glycosides, and oestrogenic substances. Sage is widely used for its astringent, stimulant, nerve strengthening, diuretic, expectorant, memory boosting, calming, anti-inflammatory, antimicrobial, antioxidant properties. It can also help with swellings, cuts, sprains, cramps, mouth ulcers, sore throat, dyspepsia, abdominal discomfort, menopausal symptoms and joint pain. Sage should be avoided throughout pregnancy and the nursing period.

Planting time and harvesting: The germination rates for sage seed are very poor, so it is best to buy ready grown plants from a garden centre and transplant them. Sage prefers a sunny, well-drained location but will tolerate partial shade. Add compost and peat moss to the soil to make a light soil mix. Dig holes big enough to accommodate the root ball of the plants, spacing them 60-90 cm apart. Loosen the roots and place each plant in a hole. Fill with soil up to the base and push down to secure. Be sure to plant at least 2 or 3 plants to have enough sage to harvest, dry and use throughout winter. Keep the soil moist for at least 7 days after planting until the new plants are established. Mulch around the base of the plants to retain moisture. Once established, let the soil dry out before watering. Nip off the flowers when they appear or the plant will cease to grow.

Harvest newly planted sage at the end of July and dry the leaves for future use. Do not harvest again, until the following June and again in August. To harvest, pluck the stems down to half-way down the plant; bunch together and hang them to dry in a well-ventilated area away from direct sun.

Part used: Leaves, oil.

Preparation: Sage is used as condiment and for flavouring food, especially when the foods are difficult to digest, are fat- or protein-rich like meat, stuffing and sauces, etc. It also makes a delicious herbal tea.

Thyme – *Thymus vulgaris*

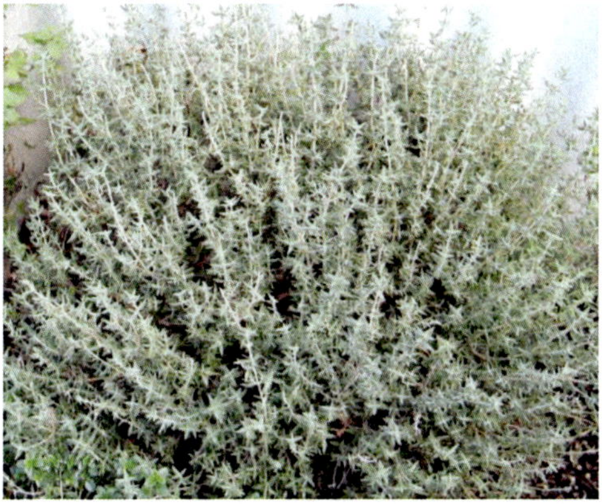

Copyright © 2005 Donovan Govan

Thyme is a hardy perennial member of the *Lamiaceae* family and is native to the Mediterranean. Its beautiful flowers are white to purple.

Properties and medicinal uses: Thyme is carminative, antioxidant, antispasmodic, anti-rheumatic, antiseptic, antiviral, diuretic, emmenagogue, expectorant, astringent, and anthelmintic.

It is commonly used in different forms for the relief of aches and pains, acne, arthritis, asthma, boils, bronchitis, bruises, burns, catarrh, cellulite, colds, coughs, cuts, cystitis, dermatitis, diarrhoea, dyspepsia, eczema, flatulence, gout, gum infections, hypotension, infectious diseases, insect bites, laryngitis, lice, oedema, oily skin, poor circulation, scabies, sinusitis, sore throat, sprains, strains, tonsillitis, and urethritis.

Planting time and harvesting: Thyme thrives best in full sun and well-drained light soil that is not too rich in nutrients (a rockery is ideal). The germination rates for thyme seed are slow and unpredictable, so it is best to buy ready grown plants from a garden centre and transplant them. Plant them out when all threat of frost has passed and the soil is warm, and space them at least 30 cm apart.

Thyme requires very little attention. Water only in very dry conditions and feed sparingly. Mulch with organic matter around October; this will protect it from severe frost and supply most of its feeding needs. Cut the plants back after they flower in summer to promote growth.

Harvest lightly (if at all) in the first year.

Part used: Leaves, oil.

Preparation: Wash well. Thyme is used to add flavour to salads, sauces, soups, stews, stuffing, meat, and poultry. It can also be used to make herbal tea, a mouth wash or gargle by infusing a handful of fresh leaves or 1 tsp of dry leaves, in boiling water. Cover for 10-15 minutes and drink or gargle when needed.

Thyme essential oil is frequently used in Aromatherapy treatments to aid digestion.

Watercress – *Nasturtium officinale*

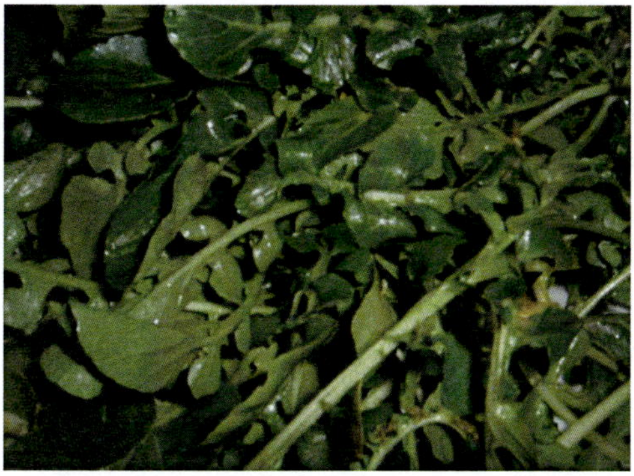

Copyright © 2009 Masparasol

Watercress is an aquatic, perennial member of the *Brassicaceae* family and native to Europe. The plants grow partially submerged under water and produce small white flowers in summer.

Properties and medicinal uses: Watercress is an excellent source of iron, copper, manganese, carotenes, calcium and folic acid as well as vitamins A, B1, B2, B6, C, and E. It is an antibacterial, diuretic, expectorant, stimulant, digestive, stomachic, antiseptic, antioxidant, and tonic.

Watercress has anticancer properties; in addition it improves the memory and mental function, cleanses the blood, lowers cholesterol and blood pressure, promotes good eyesight, cures bleeding gums, strengthens bones and teeth, and freshens the breath.

Planting time and harvesting: Watercress can be grown from seed. Plant the seeds indoors in plastic pots using a rich seed starting soil and keep the soil moist. Once the seedlings are big enough to handle (usually in April or May), transplant them into larger plastic pots with drainage holes. Place these pots in an even larger container, suitable for holding water. Sink the whole thing in the surface of the garden soil and fill the bottom container with fresh water. As the watercress grows, remember to top up the container with fresh water on a frequent basis. Once the plant has flowered, the leaves and stems are too bitter to eat, so harvest them before blooming. They will keep in the fridge for several days.

Part used: Leaves, stem.

Preparation: Wash well. Watercress is used in salads and as a garnish and also makes a lovely soup.

Yarrow – *Achillea millefolium*

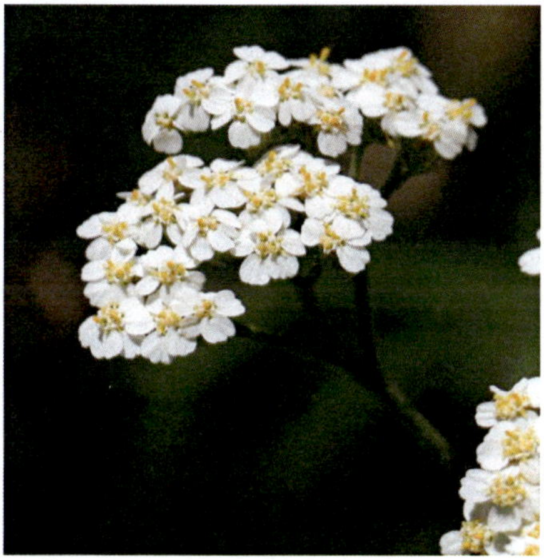

Copyright © 2010 dcrjsr

Yarrow is a flowering perennial plant in the *Asteracea* family and is native to Europe and Asia. When cultivated as a companion plant, it improves the health of other plants in the vicinity and boosts their essential oil content, making them more resistant to insects.

Properties and medicinal uses: The main constituents of yarrow are volatile oils such as linalool, camphor, sabinene, chamazulene, sesquiterpene lactones, flavonoids, alkaloids including achilleine, polyacetylenes, triterpenes, salicylic acid, coumarins, and tannins. Yarrow is an antiseptic, antispasmodic, astringent, carminative, diaphoretic, digestive, emmenagogue, stimulant, tonic, vasodilator and vulnerary. It is used to combat colds, cramps, fevers, kidney disorders, toothaches, skin irritations, haemorrhages, and to regulate menses, stimulate the flow of bile, and purify blood. When taken as a herbal tea, it is a good remedy for colds and flu, stomach ulcers, amenorrhea, abdominal cramps, abscesses, trauma and bleeding, and to reduce inflammation. Despite its many medicinal properties, large or frequent doses taken over a long period of time may cause the skin to become more sensitive to sunlight.

Planting time and harvesting: Yarrow prefers full sun and thrives best in well-drained soil. Sow the seeds indoors in moist potting compost, about 6-8 weeks before the last frost. Cover the seeds very lightly with more compost and place the pots in a warm sunny location. The seeds will germinate in 14-21 days, depending on the conditions. You may wish to speed up this process by covering the top of the pot with plastic wrap to retain moisture and heat, removing the wrap once the seeds have sprouted. Transplant the seedlings when they grow large enough to handle, after gradually exposing them to more light and outdoor temperatures. Dig a hole large enough to take the roots, spacing plants 30-45 cm apart. Gently firm the soil around each plant base and ensure all foliage is above ground. Water in well. After planting, water only very occasionally. Yarrow plants will rot if over-watered.

Harvest when the plant is dry and in full bloom. Cut the stems and flowers in the morning. Dry them by tying the stems together and hanging them upside down in a dry, dark, well-ventilated place. Once dried, store foliage and flowers separately in airtight containers for later use.

Part used: Flowering tops, leaves, essential oil.

Preparation: The younger leaves make a pleasant leaf vegetable when cooked as spinach, or added to soup. Yarrow is sweet with a slightly bitter taste, so is not to everyone's taste. The leaves can also be dried and used as a herb in cooking. To make herbal tea, add 1 tsp of dried yarrow to 1 cup boiling water, steep for 10 minutes and sweeten to taste.

SUPERFOODS

Superfoods are foods with a high phytonutrient content. Their health benefits lie in the fact that they contain significant amounts of antioxidants, which prevent or slow down oxidative damage in the body. Oxidative damage contributes towards many major diseases of the body including heart disease, diabetes, and cancer. Antioxidants seek out the free radicals and prevent and repair the damage caused by them.

Sprouted seeds

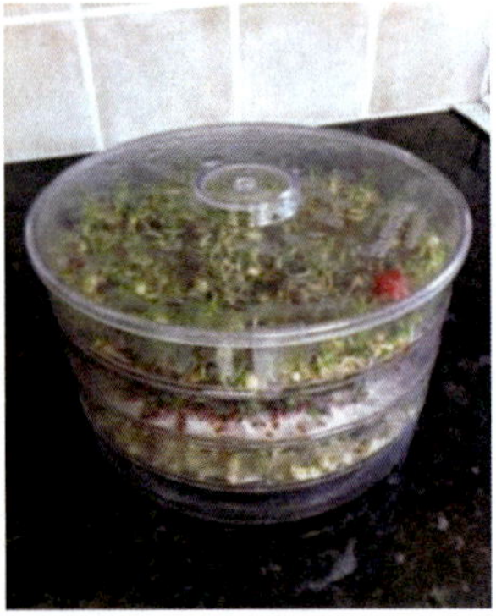

Sprouted seeds are so easy to grow and are absolutely packed with nutrients. They contain very high concentrations of proteins, minerals, enzymes, trace elements and vitamins, as well as fibre to regulate the digestive system. And as they are only picked at the last moment to add to a dish, virtually no valuable nutrients are lost prior to consumption.

Sprouted seeds can be grown in your kitchen (see **How to Grow Your Own Produce** on page 157). Just get yourself some seeds and a sprouter (see **Useful Links** on page 317), and in no time you'll be producing your own healthy organic food!

Purple sweet potato

This purple sweet potato is grown for its anti-cancer, anti-ageing and antioxidant properties. Its purple colouring is responsible for the amount of anthocyanin in the potato, which lowers the risk of cancer and could even slow down certain types of the disease. In tests, scientists used anthocyanin to treat colon cancer and found the pigment slowed down the growth of cancerous cells.

Sun chlorella

Chlorella is a type of green algae. Whilst research suggests that Chlorella could be effective in fighting major diseases, it has been shown to reduce body-fat percentage and blood-glucose levels and help those with type 2 diabetes, obesity and heart disease. It boosts the immune system, is an energiser, a digestive aid, helps fight depression and detoxifies the body.

Chlorella is very rich in protein and contains nine essential amino acids, as well as vitamins and minerals. It is safe for most people to take, with the exception of those who are taking blood thinning medications. This is because chlorella contains vitamin K1, a vitamin that is important in helping the blood to clot, which opposes the medication's anticoagulant action. Chlorella is available in tablet form.

Wheatgrass

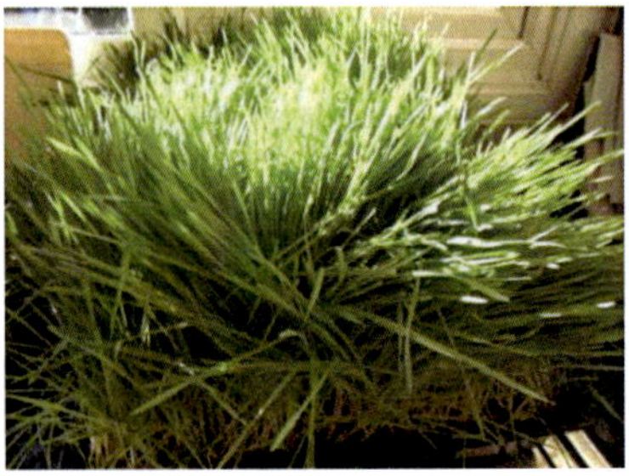

Wheatgrass juice contains almost everything necessary to fuel the body. It is commonly believed that in order to supply the body with protein we should eat protein. However, this is not true. The body uses amino acids to build protein; so when we eat protein, e.g. grains, pulses, fish, meat, the body has to break down these proteins into amino acids and then reconstitute them into the required proteins. By providing the body with the amino acids to produce the protein it needs, the process of breaking down protein in meat, etc is avoided, which is especially good if that protein has been damaged by cooking.

Wheatgrass juice is renowned for its healing properties. Due to its concentrated source of chlorophyll and other nutrients, just 2 oz provides the same nourishment as up to 4lbs of fresh green vegetables. It is an excellent energiser, blood tonic, has natural antibiotic properties, and helps maintain a healthy digestive tract. Wheatgrass juice is also a powerful antioxidant.

Grow your own wheatgrass

Soak 500g wheatgrass seeds in water for 8 hours. Just before they finish soaking, prepare a 40 cm x 20 cm seed tray, with a depth of 5 cm, by adding 2.5 cm of moist organic compost and potting mix. After soaking, drain the seeds, rinse thoroughly and drain them again.

Spread the seeds evenly over the compost mix. Add another 13 mm of soil and then water in using a watering can with a rose. The soil should be moist but not soaking. It is important to keep the soil moist whilst the wheatgrass is growing, so water the tray every day. Cover the tray with another tray, or plastic bubble-wrap to help to keep in the moisture.

Approximately 3 days later the wheatgrass will be about 5 cm in height. You can then remove the cover from the tray and place the tray in a position where the wheatgrass will receive plenty of indirect sunlight. (Do not place the wheatgrass in direct sunlight as this will dry out the soil, inhibiting growth.) Sunlight enables the wheatgrass to produce chlorophyll, transforming it from yellow to a vibrant green.

Harvest when the wheatgrass is about 15-20 cm in height as this is when it is at its nutritional best. To harvest, simply trim a centimetre or two above the soil surface using scissors or a chef's knife. Rinse the wheatgrass thoroughly before juicing it.

Once the seed cover is removed, you can harvest the wheatgrass over a period of 4-5 days. This can be increased or decreased by changing the temperature and light levels in the place where the wheatgrass is situated. 18-20° C is ideal for growing wheatgrass. If the air is too hot or humid then mould can occur (this looks like white blobs, which form around the base of the wheatgrass stalks when it is alive and black spots when it is dead). If mould does form, trim the wheatgrass well above the mould to avoid ingesting it. Some people are allergic to mould and it is also bad for those suffering from asthma. Ingesting mould can cause instant reactions like headaches, nausea and hives. If your crop does get mould, remember to sterilize the tray before using it for the next crop.

If you harvest more wheatgrass than you need, place the excess in an airtight container and refrigerate. This way, the wheatgrass should keep for a few days.

Once accustomed to the time cycle involved in growing wheatgrass, the amount of juice a tray yields, and how much wheatgrass juice you consume a day, you will be able to plan when to plant the next tray of wheatgrass to ensure a constant supply. Growing your own wheatgrass is the most economical way of obtaining a regular intake of this amazing superfood. Start by drinking approximately 1 oz of wheatgrass juice a day. Increase this to 2 oz a day after a few weeks, gradually building up to 4 oz. Remember, wheatgrass is gluten free. Although wheat *grain* contains gluten, wheat*grass* does not.

It is not recommended that you re-grow the wheatgrass after its first harvesting period. A great deal of nutritional value comes from the seed as it sprouts and is contained within the first harvest. A second harvest would contain far less nutrition. As well as the loss of nutritional content, re-growing the wheatgrass increases the chance of mould.

Spinach

Spinach is one of the best sources of lutein, which offers significant protection against age-related conditions. It is also a good source of iron. Spinach contains high amounts of the antioxidants glutathione and alpha-lipoic acid. Together they help detoxify the cells and protect both aqueous and lipid media throughout the body. Although alpha-lipoic acid is naturally produced in low levels in the body, with age it produces less.

Turmeric root

Turmeric also has amazing antioxidant properties. It boosts the activity of one of the most important detoxifying enzymes in the body, glutathione S-transferase. Studies show that the antioxidant activity of turmeric exceeds that of vitamin E and beta-carotene. The most commonly known antioxidants are:

Antioxidant	**Found in**
Vitamin A and carotenoids	Carrots, squash, broccoli, sweet potatoes, tomatoes, kale, collards, cantaloupe, peaches, apricots
Vitamin C	Citrus fruits, green peppers, broccoli, green leafy vegetables, strawberries, tomatoes
Vitamin E	Nuts, seeds, whole grains, green leafy vegetables, vegetable oil, liver oil
Selenium	Fish, shellfish, red meat, grains, eggs, chicken, garlic

Flavonoids / polyphenols	Soya, red wine, purple grapes, pomegranate, cranberries
Lycopene	Tomato, tomato products, pink grapefruit, watermelon
Lutein	Kale, broccoli, kiwi, brussels sprouts, spinach
Lignan	Flax seed, oatmeal, barley, rye

Beans, grain products, fruits and vegetables are all rich sources of antioxidants. It is best to obtain antioxidants from foods instead of supplements.

VITAMINS, MINERALS, FATTY ACIDS & AMINO ACIDS

Below is a list of vitamins, minerals, fatty acids and amino acids. I have included their health benefits, dietary sources, signs of deficiency and side effects in order to give a well-rounded view of each nutrient. However, although in some cases the side effects may seem a little alarming, please remember that it is very difficult to overdose on any vitamin, mineral, fatty acid or amino acid when eating a sensible diet, as advocated in the previous pages.

Please note that this information is for guidance only.

VITAMINS

Fat soluble vitamins

Fat-soluble vitamins are absorbed, along with fat from the intestine, into the circulation. Once absorbed into the circulation, they are then carried to the liver to be stored. Anyone with a disorder that affects the absorption of fat could have a deficiency of these vitamins.

Water soluble vitamins

Water-soluble vitamins are stored in the body for only a short time and are then expelled by the kidneys. The only exception is vitamin B12, which gets stored in the liver. For optimal health, water-soluble vitamins need to be consumed daily.

Vitamin A (aka: carotene, retinol) – fat soluble

Health benefits: Vitamin A promotes good eye health, the development of bones and teeth, regulation of the immune system, and assists white blood cells to fight infection. It is also an antioxidant, which helps prevent and repair damage in the body caused by free radicals.

Sources: Apricots, asparagus, beetroot, broccoli, butternut squash, cantaloupe melon, carrots, cod liver oil, dandelion greens, eggs, garlic, kale, mustard, peaches, spinach, sweet potatoes, and pumpkin.

Deficiency can lead to: Night blindness; dry, scaly skin; loss of appetite; anaemia; kidney stones.

Side effects: High levels of vitamin A in the body can lead to headaches, vomiting, abnormalities of the liver, loss of bone density, birth defects, vertigo, and disorders of the nervous system. However, this is unlikely to be caused by a sensible diet, but rather from taking large amounts of vitamin A in supplement form.

Vitamin B1 (aka: thiamin) – water soluble

Health benefits: All B vitamins help maintain muscle tone inside the digestive tract, and encourage a healthy nervous system, skin, eyes, mouth and liver. Vitamin B1 helps convert blood sugar into energy, improves the circulation, maintains healthy mucous membranes, and supports the heart, nervous system and muscles.

Sources: Dried beans, brown rice, cereals, chicken, egg yolks, fish, peanuts, peas, soya beans, wheat germ, whole grains and yeast.

Deficiency can lead to: Tiredness, irritability, loss of appetite, muscle wastage, mental illness, anorexia, enlarged heart, nerve changes, abnormal heart rhythm.

Side effects: Vitamin B1 is not harmful as part of a sensible diet; however, very high levels in supplement form may cause drowsiness.

Vitamin B2 (aka: riboflavin) – water soluble

Health benefits: All B vitamins help maintain muscle tone inside the digestive tract, and encourage a healthy nervous system, skin, eyes, mouth and liver. Vitamin B2 boosts the immune system and helps in cases of anaemia, cataracts, migraine, Parkinson's Disease, pre-eclampsia, and sickle cell anaemia.

Sources: Asparagus, avocados, beans, broccoli, brussels sprouts, cereals, cheese, chicken, currants, eggs, fish, fruit, nuts and spinach.

Deficiency can lead to: Painful tongue, cracks at mouth corners, chapped lips, sore throat, skin rash.

Side effects: None. Any excess amounts of vitamin B2 are naturally expelled from the body within a few days.

Vitamin B3 (aka: niacin) – water soluble

Health benefits: All B vitamins help maintain muscle tone inside the digestive tract, and encourage a healthy nervous system, skin, eyes, mouth and liver. Vitamin B3 helps rid the body of harmful chemicals, improves circulation, and balances good and bad cholesterol levels. It also relieves stress, promotes good heart health, encourages DNA repair, and reduces inflammation in painful joints.

Sources: Broccoli, carrots, corn flour, eggs, fish, potatoes, tomatoes, and wholewheat.

Deficiency can lead to: Slow metabolism, diarrhoea, dermatitis, dementia, sore mouth and tongue, digestive problems, amnesia, delirium.

Side effects: As part of a healthy diet, vitamin B3 is not harmful. However, high doses can interact with certain medications and should only be taken under the direction of a qualified healthcare provider as it can cause skin flushes, liver damage, and stomach ulcers. Vitamin B3 supplements should not be taken by anyone suffering with gout.

Vitamin B5 (aka: pantothenic acid) – water soluble

Health benefits: All B vitamins help maintain muscle tone inside the digestive tract, and encourage a healthy nervous system, skin, eyes, mouth and liver. Vitamin B5 supports the adrenal gland, releases energy, aids in the metabolism of fat, protein and carbohydrates, helps create lipids, neurotransmitters, haemoglobin and steroid hormones, and antibodies.

Sources: Most foods, especially beans, eggs, salt water fish, fresh vegetables, wholewheat.

Deficiency can lead to: Deficiency of vitamin B5 is extremely rare. However, symptoms include irritability, fatigue, apathy, numbness, muscle cramps, hypoglycaemia.

Side effects: As part of a healthy diet, vitamin B5 is not harmful. However, excessive amounts can cause diarrhoea.

Vitamin B6 (aka: pyridoxine, pyridoxamine, pyridoxal) – water soluble

Health benefits: All B vitamins help maintain muscle tone inside the digestive tract, and encourage a healthy nervous system, skin, eyes, mouth and liver. Vitamin B6 reduces oedema, aids in the absorption of fats, helps maintain sodium and potassium balance, and promotes red blood cell formation.

Sources: Carrots, chicken, eggs, fish, peas, spinach, soya beans, sunflower seeds, walnuts, and whole grains.

Deficiency can lead to: Anaemia, convulsions, cracks at mouth corners, dermatitis, nausea, confusion.

Side effects: Neurological abnormalities if consumed in excessively high quantities.

Vitamin B7 (aka: biotin) – water soluble

Health benefits: All B vitamins help maintain muscle tone inside the digestive tract, and encourage a healthy nervous system, skin, eyes, mouth and liver. Vitamin B7 aids cell growth, fatty acid production, the metabolism of carbohydrates, fats and proteins, and promotes healthy hair and nails.

Sources: Almonds, bananas, brewer's yeast, cauliflower, eggs, filberts, grapefruit, mushrooms, salmon, sardines, soya, strawberries, sweet potatoes, watermelon.

Deficiency can lead to: Anaemia, depression, hair loss, high blood sugar, insomnia, loss of appetite, muscular pain, nausea, sore tongue.

Side effects: None.

Vitamin B9 (aka: folic acid) – water soluble

Health benefits: All B vitamins help maintain muscle tone inside the digestive tract, and encourage a healthy nervous system, skin, eyes, mouth and liver. Vitamin B9 aids the relief of Alzheimer's disease, anaemia, bipolar disorder, cancer, cataracts, cervical dysplasia, depression, gout, heart disease, infertility, migraine, osteoarthritis, osteoporosis, psoriasis, rheumatoid arthritis, vitiligo, warts. Take before and during pregnancy to lower the risk of birth defects.

Sources: Green leafy vegetables, beans, peas, lentils, egg yolks, baker's yeast, pasta, cereal, bread, sunflower seeds, oranges, pineapples, cantaloupe, honeydew melon, grapefruit, bananas, raspberries, strawberries, beets, corn, tomatoes, vegetable juice, romaine lettuce.

Deficiency can lead to: Inflammation of the tongue, diarrhoea, depression, confusion, anaemia, and birth defects.

Side effects: None.

Vitamin B12 (cobalamin) – water soluble

Health benefits: All B vitamins help maintain muscle tone inside the digestive tract, and encourage a healthy nervous system, skin, eyes, mouth and liver. Vitamin B12 supports healthy nerve cells and red blood cells, helps in the making of DNA, and aids digestion, protein synthesis, and metabolism of carbohydrates and fats.

Sources: Clams, eggs, herring, mackerel, seafood, and tofu.

Deficiency can lead to: Pernicious anaemia.

Side effects: None.

Vitamin B15 (aka: pangamic acid) – water soluble

Health benefits: All B vitamins help maintain muscle tone inside the digestive tract, and encourage a healthy nervous system, skin, eyes, mouth and liver. There is some debate about whether vitamin B15 is actually necessary to maintain a healthy body. However, in some countries it has been used to treat excess lactic acid, muscle fatigue, alcoholism and drug addiction, senility, schizophrenia, autism, heart disease, high blood pressure, diabetes, skin disease, liver disease.

Sources: Whole grains, brown rice, brewer's yeast, pumpkin seeds, sunflower seeds.

Deficiency can lead to: Unknown.

Side effects: None.

Vitamin C (aka: ascorbic acid) – water soluble

Health benefits: Vitamin C is a powerful antioxidant, it maintains and repairs connective tissues, bones, teeth and cartilage, promotes healing and absorption of iron, lowers blood pressure, supports the nervous system, regulates blood glucose levels, aids the immune system, and assists in healing wounds.

Sources: Peppers, broccoli, spinach, brussels sprouts, citrus fruits, berries, tomatoes, potatoes, cabbage.

Deficiency can lead to: Scurvy, anaemia, loose teeth, joint pain, poor healing, hair loss, urinary stones, acid stomach, nausea, diarrhoea, headache, fatigue.

Side effects: Vitamin C is acidic and excessive intake can cause upset stomach.

Vitamin D (aka: calciferol) – fat soluble

Health benefits: Vitamin D promotes strong bones and teeth and aids calcium absorption. It helps in the fight against cancer and may help prevent Alzheimer's disease. Exposure to sunlight may reduce the risk of heart disease and diabetes in older people. Research has found that pensioners who regularly go out into the sunshine had higher levels of vitamin D than those who stay indoors. If vitamin D levels are low, it can trigger metabolic syndrome, a condition that affects the body's ability to produce insulin, significantly increasing the risk of heart disease and diabetes.

Sources: Fish oils, butter, egg yolks, sunlight, and fortified foods such as bread and cereals.

Deficiency can lead to: Rickets.

Side effects: High intake of vitamin D can result in excess absorption of calcium, potentially causing kidney stones.

Vitamin E (aka: tocopherol) – fat soluble

Health benefits: Vitamin E is another powerful antioxidant providing protection and maintenance of cellular membranes. It supports the immune system, reduces long-term risk of dementia, and helps regulate metabolism and prevent heart disease.

Sources: Vegetable oils, whole grains, nuts & seeds, green leafy vegetables, asparagus, peaches, kiwi, mango.

Deficiency can lead to: Possible muscular dystrophy, anaemia, weakness, neurological problems, muscle cramps.

Side effects: Almost unknown for side effects but in severe cases may cause excessive bleeding or formation of blood clots.

Vitamin K (aka: naphthoquinoids) – fat soluble

Health benefits: Vitamin K is a powerful antioxidant. It helps blood coagulation, assists the maintenance of strong bones, protects against heart disease, and may possibly help regulate blood sugar levels.

Sources: Kale, brussels sprouts, spinach, broccoli, cabbage, dark green lettuce, pistachio nuts.

Deficiency can lead to: Deficiency of vitamin K is very rare. However, symptoms include bleeding due to lack of clotting factors, bruising.

Side effects: Anyone taking blood thinning medications should be closely monitored by a medical practitioner as vitamin K can have an adverse effect.

MINERALS

Calcium

Health benefits: Calcium helps maintain strong bones and teeth, and controls nerve impulses and muscle contractions.

Sources: Tofu, fortified orange juice and bread, green leafy vegetables, bones in fish.

Deficiency can lead to: Bone mineral loss.

Side effects: Excessive calcium intake can lead to constipation, urinary stones, calcium deposits in soft tissues, and inhibition of mineral absorption.

Copper

Health benefits: Copper is a powerful antioxidant and anti-inflammatory. It promotes proper growth and protection of the skeletal, nervous and cardiovascular systems, helps utilize iron in the body, balances cholesterol levels, benefits the connective tissues and thyroid glands, helps control heart rhythm, eases arthritis, and promotes wound healing.

Sources: Oysters, molasses, cocoa, black pepper, lobster, nuts, sunflower seeds, green olives, avocados, and wheat bran.

Deficiency can lead to: Anaemia, brittle bones, osteoporosis, high cholesterol levels, low resistance to infections, birth defects, hypo-pigmentation, and thyroid disorders.

Side effects: Side effects from copper are very rare but excessive copper intake can cause nausea, vomiting, stomach ache, headache, dizziness, weakness, diarrhoea, and a metallic taste in the mouth.

Fluoride

Health benefits: Fluoride helps maintain healthy tooth and bone structure.

Sources: Tap water, tea, and marine fish eaten with bones.

Deficiency can lead to: Tooth decay.

Side effects: Excessive fluoride can lead to increased bone density, mottling of teeth, impaired kidney function.

Iodine

Health benefits: Iodine is an essential part of thyroid hormones, which are needed for the regulation of metabolism.

Sources: Sea salt, seafood.

Deficiency can lead to: Goitre (enlarged thyroid), cretinism (birth defect).

Side effects: Excessive iodine intake can lead to depression of thyroid activity, hyperthyroidism.

Iron

Health benefits: Iron is important for the formation of haemoglobin and helps transport oxygen to the blood cells. It aids good muscle and brain function, helps regulate body temperature, strengthens the immune system, improves concentration and fights fatigue.

Sources: Legumes, lentils, soya beans, green leafy vegetables, whole grains, cereals, bread, turnip and dried fruits. (N.B. Foods containing vitamin C will help the absorption of iron in the body.)

Deficiency can lead to: Fatigue, anaemia.

Side effects: Excessive amounts of iron can lead the production of free radicals, which are harmful to the body.

Magnesium

Health benefits: Magnesium helps with the transmission of nerve impulses, energy transfer, and the activation of many enzymes.

Sources: Grains, legumes, nuts, seeds, green vegetables, and mineral water.

Deficiency can lead to: Neurological disturbances, cardiovascular problems, kidney disorders, nausea, poor growth.

Side effects: Excessive magnesium intake can cause nausea, vomiting, diarrhoea, impaired central nervous system.

Manganese

Health benefits: Manganese is a powerful antioxidant, which helps fight harmful free radicals. It promotes healthy bones and good brain function, regulates blood sugar levels, alleviates PMT, aids vitamin absorption in the body, and maintains function of the digestive system.

Sources: Raspberries, strawberries, blackberries, tropical fruits, pineapples, bananas, grapes, garlic, beetroot, green beans, rice, peppermint, oats, nuts, watercress, lettuce, cucumber, carrots, leeks, spinach, molasses, cloves, turmeric, tofu, figs, and whole wheat.

Deficiency can lead to: High blood pressure, heart problems, muscle cramps, malformed bones, high cholesterol, poor eyesight, hearing loss, and memory loss.

Side effects: Excess manganese disrupts the absorption of dietary iron. Long-term excess levels may result in anaemia.

Phosphorus

Health benefits: Phosphorus is essential for the growth and maintenance of strong bones, and energy transfer in the cells.

Sources: Phosphorus is found in practically all foods.

Deficiency can lead to: Weakness, bone loss, kidney disorders, cardio-respiratory failure.

Side effects: Excessive phosphorus intake can lead to a drop in blood calcium levels, and calcium deposits in soft tissue.

Potassium

Health benefits: Potassium is vital for good nerve function and to maintain the body water balance.

Sources: Fruits, vegetables, grains, legumes.

Deficiency can lead to: Muscular weakness, nausea, drowsiness, paralysis, confusion, disruption of cardiac rhythm.

Side effects: Excessive potassium intake can lead to cardiac arrest.

Selenium

Health benefits: Selenium helps protect the cells from oxidative damage, and aids immune response.

Sources: Seafood, meat, eggs, whole grains.

Deficiency can lead to: Muscle pain and weakness, heart disorders.

Side effects: Excessive selenium intake can lead to hair loss, nausea and vomiting, weakness and irritability.

Sodium

Health benefits: Sodium aids body water balance, acid-base balance, and nerve functions.

Sources: Salt, soy sauce, salted foods.

Deficiency can lead to: Muscle weakness, loss of appetite, nausea, vomiting; however, sodium deficiency is rare.

Side effects: Large amounts of sodium can lead to oedema, hypertension.

Zinc

Health benefits: Zinc aids in the synthesis of proteins, RNA and DNA; wound healing; immune response, and the ability to taste.

Sources: Whole grains, eggs, seafood (especially oysters).

Deficiency can lead to: Growth failure, loss of appetite, impaired taste, skin rash, impaired immune functions, poor wound healing.

Side effects: Excessive amounts of zinc can lead to vomiting, impaired immune function, decline in blood HDL levels, and impaired copper absorption.

FATTY ACIDS

α-Linolenic acid (the shortest chain omega-3 fatty acid)

Health benefits: Anti-clotting effect, lowers risk of coronary heart disease and atherosclerosis, lowers the level of fats in the blood, lowers high blood pressure, lowers high cholesterol, stimulates blood circulation, assists immune function, improves memory and learning skills, alleviates arthritis due to its anti-inflammatory properties, prevents allergies in children (if taken during pregnancy), and promotes healthy skin, nails and hair.

Sources: Flaxseeds, flaxseed oil, rapeseed oil, soya beans and soya bean oil, pumpkin seeds and pumpkin seed oil, tofu, walnuts and walnut oil.

Deficiency can lead to: Scaly skin, hair loss and slow wound healing.

Side effects: None. However, anyone taking blood thinning medications or cholesterol lowering medications should consult their doctor regarding their intake of omega-3.

Linoleic acid (the shortest chain omega-6 fatty acid)

Health benefits: Omega-6 is believed to lower blood pressure, relieve menopausal and PMT symptoms, and reduce bone loss.

Sources: Pistachios, almonds, walnuts, sesame seeds, watermelon seeds, sunflower seeds, flax seeds, cashews, brazil nuts, pine nuts, peanuts, pecans, pumpkin seeds and hazelnuts.

Deficiency can lead to: Scaly skin, hair loss and slow wound healing.

Side effects: Excessive amounts of omega-6 can lead to depression, attention deficiency disorder, weight gain, obesity, poor sleep patterns, cancers, and arthritis.

AMINO ACIDS

Isoleucine

Health benefits: Isoleucine is necessary for the production of haemoglobin, encourages clotting at site of injury, heals and repairs muscle tissue, regulates blood sugar levels, and increases stamina.

Sources: Nuts, seeds, chicken, eggs, fish, lentils, peas, soya.

Deficiency can lead to: Headaches, dizziness, fatigue, depression, confusion, and irritability.

Side effects: None. However, people with kidney or liver disease should not consume high intakes of amino acids without medical advice.

Lysine

Health benefits: Lysine promotes collagen formation for healthy bones, cartilage, ligaments, and tendons, aids calcium absorption, and supports the immune system.

Sources: Poultry, cod, sardines, legumes, nuts, eggs, soya beans, spirulina, fenugreek seed, and brewer's yeast.

Deficiency can lead to: Loss of energy, loss of appetite, inability to concentrate, hair loss, and bloodshot eyes. Lysine deficiency can also cause anaemia, reproductive disorders, and delayed growth.

Side effects: Very rare, but abdominal cramps and diarrhoea have been reported.

Leucine

Health benefits: Leucine regulates blood sugar, prevents muscle breakdown, heals bones and skin, increases energy, and aids weight loss by increasing the metabolic rate during exercise.

Sources: Eggs, poultry, shrimp, black beans, yogurt, cottage cheese, and legumes.

Deficiency can lead to: Headaches, dizziness, depression, fatigue, confusion and irritability.

Side effects: None. However, people with depression, liver or kidney disease should consult their G.P. regarding safe intake levels.

Methionine

Health benefits: Methionine helps the body process and eliminate fat, build healthy tissues and promotes cardiovascular health. It also helps reduce the level of inflammatory histamines in the body.

Sources: Beans, eggs, fish, garlic, lentils, onions, soya beans, seeds, and yogurt.

Deficiency can lead to: Lethargy, oedema, liver damage, muscle loss, fat loss, skin lesions, and weakness.

Side effects: None.

Phenylalanine

Health benefits: Essential for good growth and functioning of the central nervous system.

Sources: Fish, poultry, eggs, yogurt, tofu, soya beans and soya products

Deficiency can lead to: Lack of appetite, memory loss, lack of concentration, lethargy, confusion, stunted growth, and muscle weakness.

Side effects: Excessive intake of phenylalanine can cause nerve damage. Sufferers of high blood pressure or migraines, and those taking antidepressants should consult their G.P. regarding healthy levels.

Threonine

Health benefits: Threonine promotes production of collagen, elastin and muscle tissue, builds strong bones and teeth, supports cardiovascular, liver, central nervous system and immune system function.

Sources: Grains, mushrooms, and leafy green vegetables.

Deficiency can lead to: Agitation, confusion, digestion difficulties and fatty liver

Side effects: Excess threonine can lead to ammonia toxicity.

Tryptophan

Health benefits: Tryptophan soothes nerves and anxiety, enhances relaxation and sleep, relieves minor symptoms of PMT, and reduces carbohydrate cravings. Tryptophan is important for the production of serotonin, one of the key brain chemicals involved in regulating mood.

Sources: Oats, bananas, dried dates, cottage cheese, fish, turkey, peanuts. Lower concentrations found in corn, cereal grains, legumes, eggs, some nuts and seeds.

Deficiency can lead to: Depression, insomnia, schizophrenia, suicidal thoughts, carbohydrate cravings.

Side effects: Excess levels of tryptophan can lead to agitation, confusion, diarrhoea, fever, overactive reflexes, poor coordination, restlessness, shivering, sweating, trembling, twitching, and vomiting. People taking serotonin increasing medication should consult their G.P. regarding safe levels.

Valine

Health benefits: Valine promotes normal growth, repairs tissues, regulates blood sugar, and provides the body with energy. It also helps stimulate the central nervous system, and aids proper mental functioning.

Sources: Mushrooms, peanuts, and soya protein.

Deficiency can lead to: Maple syrup urine disease (MSUD), caused by the inability to metabolize leucine, isoleucine, and valine, and causing the urine to smell like maple syrup. A deficiency of valine may also affect the myelin covering of the nerves, and cause degenerative neurological conditions.

Side effects: Excessively high intake of valine may cause a skin crawling sensation and hallucinations, disrupt liver and kidney function and increase ammonia in the body. People with impaired liver or kidney function should consult their G.P. regarding safe levels.

TOP TIPS

How to store fresh herbs

- Snip off the bottom of the stems.
- The leaves must be completely dry. Do not rinse the herbs until you need to use them.
- Partially fill a jar or glass with water and place the stem ends of the herbs into the water.
- If you wish to store the herbs in the refrigerator, cover them loosely with a plastic bag. Most herbs store well in the refrigerator; however, basil prefers to be stored at room temperature as it is susceptible to cold.
- Change the water as soon as it starts to discolour.

Fresh herbs will last 2 weeks or longer when stored in this way.

How to keep green vegetables crisp

Boil an inch of hot water with a pinch of salt in a covered saucepan. Once boiling, drop in the vegetables and replace the lid. Drain after three minutes and rinse the vegetables under running cold water to take the heat out and keep them crisp and green.

With vegetables such as asparagus, you can stand the stalks up straight in a jar of water and cover the tips with a plastic bag. Leave in the coldest part of the refrigerator for no more than 2 days.

For juices

When making batches of vegetable juice over several days, store washed carrots and stalks of celery in containers full of water in the refrigerator.

You can also keep lettuce leaves spread out and stored vertically in a container with layers of paper towel in between each leaf to help absorb any excess moisture. Fresh lettuce will last a week or more when stored this way.

Onions

Never keep a portion of left-over raw onion (not even wrapped and put in the fridge). Once cut, onions are like a magnet for bacteria and are often the cause of food poisoning. If you cannot use the whole onion at once, the left-over portion should be discarded.

USEFUL LINKS

If you'd like to obtain any items mentioned in this book, it is possible to find most of them online. I've added the following links to get you started.

JUICERS

Most juicers are ideal for use with the majority of foodstuffs; however, not all juicers can juice wheatgrass and other leafy green vegetables, e.g. parsley or coriander, successfully. For this you need a masticating juicer, which is available from various companies online including the following:

http://www.wheatgrass-uk.com/shop/
http://www.juiceland.co.uk/
http://www.energiseyourlife.com/
http://www.happyjuicer.com/

SPROUTERS

Growing your own healthy, nutritious sprouts is very simple. Whichever model of sprouter you choose the process of sprouting is the same and, used correctly, the sprouts will be of the same high quality. To see what's available, take a look at the following sites.

www.avogel.co.uk/
http://www.wheatgrass-uk.com/shop/
http://www.seedsofsustainability.org/
http://www.beansandherbs.co.uk/sendagift.htm

FOOD DEHYDRATORS

If you'd like to control the quality of the food you eat, save money, make the most of seasonal foods, take advantage of special offers at the supermarket, and help the environment by cutting down on packaging, then a food dehydrator could be the answer. Check out the links below.

http://www.juiceland.co.uk/cat--Food-Dehydrator-Guide--dehydrating.html
http://www.excaliburdehydrator.com

A. VOGEL HERBAL REMEDIES

Alfred Vogel, the natural health pioneer, established his company in 1963 to produce his fresh A.Vogel herbal remedies. As Alfred Vogel found decades ago, many factors influence the quality of a herbal remedy, which is why we still choose to use freshly harvested plants when making most of the range. Today A.Vogel remains a leading European manufacturer of fresh herbal remedies, such as the well-known Echinaforce.

www.avogel.co.uk
Tel: 01294 277344

SUN CHLORELLA

For over 40 years Sun Chlorella has been at the forefront of research and development of chlorella, a wonderful natural wholefood. Sun Chlorella® "A" tablets are the best-selling chlorella supplements in Japan. Their unique patented process pulverises the cell walls to release the valuable nutrients within, including chlorophyll for detoxing, and a whole range of important vitamins and minerals such as B12, D, Beta-Carotene, Folic Acid, Iron and essential amino acids.

https://www.sunchlorella.co.uk/

ACONBURY SPROUTS

Based in rural Herefordshire, Aconbury Sprouts have been growing the very best organic sprouted seeds and beans since 1985 and are passionate about tasty nutritious foods. Their online store offers fresh wheatgrass and greens as well as everything you need to grow and sprout at home. You'll find them at:

http://www.wheatgrass-uk.com/shop/
Tel: 01981 241336

THE HERB SOCIETY

The Herb Society

Over eighty years as the UK's leading society for increasing the understanding, use and appreciation of herbs and their benefits to health.

The Herb Society is an internationally-renowned educational charity dedicated to encouraging the appreciation and use of herbs, bringing together those interested in herbs whether they are professionals or amateurs. Their website contains a mine of information for anyone interested in the health properties of herbs.

http://www.herbsociety.org.uk/